INTANGIBLES

INTANGIBLES

The
UNEXPECTED
Traits *of*
HIGH-PERFORMING
Healthcare Leaders

Amer Kaissi

ACHE Management Series

Your board, staff, or clients may also benefit from this book's insight. For more information on quantity discounts, contact the Health Administration Press Marketing Manager at (312) 424-9450.

This publication is intended to provide accurate and authoritative information in regard to the subject matter covered. It is sold, or otherwise provided, with the understanding that the publisher is not engaged in rendering professional services. If professional advice or other expert assistance is required, the services of a competent professional should be sought.

The statements and opinions contained in this book are strictly those of the author and do not represent the official positions of the American College of Healthcare Executives or the Foundation of the American College of Healthcare Executives.

22 21   5   4   3

Library of Congress Cataloging-in-Publication Data
Title: Intangibles : the unexpected traits of high-performing healthcare
    leaders / Amer A. Kaissi.
Description: Chicago, IL : HAP, [2017] | Series: ACHE management series |
    Includes bibliographical references.
Identifiers: LCCN 2017020312 | ISBN 9781567939255 (alk. paper) | ISBN
    9781567939262 (ebook) | ISBN 9781567939279 (xml) | ISBN 9781567939286
    (epub) | ISBN 9781567939293 (mobi)
Subjects: LCSH: Health services administration. | Leadership.
Classification: LCC RA971.K26 2017 | DDC 362.10683—dc23 LC record available at https://
lccn.loc.gov/2017020312

The paper used in this publication meets the minimum requirements of American National Standard for Information Sciences—Permanence of Paper for Printed Library Materials, ANSI Z39.48-1984. ∞ ™

Acquisitions editor: Jennette E. McClain; Project manager: Theresa L. Rothschadl; Cover designer: Brad Norr; Layout: PerfecType

Found an error or a typo? We want to know! Please e-mail it to hapbooks@ache.org, mentioning the book's title and putting "Book Error" in the subject line.

For photocopying and copyright information, please contact Copyright Clearance Center at www.copyright.com or at (978) 750-8400.

Health Administration Press
A division of the Foundation of the American
    College of Healthcare Executives
300 S. Riverside Plaza, Suite 1900
Chicago, Illinois 60606-6698
(312) 424-2800

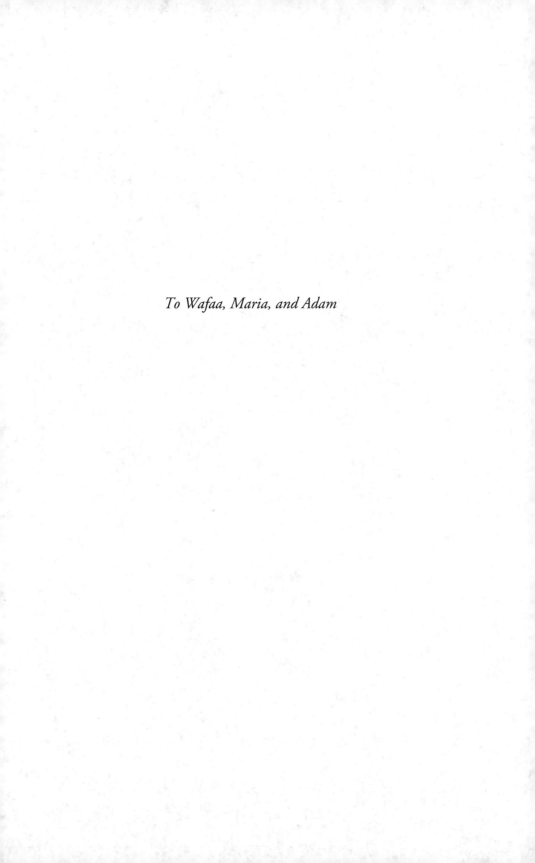

To Wafaa, Maria, and Adam

Contents

Foreword

ONE OF THE most difficult challenges related to corporate leadership is dealing with change. Change is the single constant in organizations. Change will occur whether you are standing still or growing organically or by consolidation. Organizations that adapt to change will be the survivors.

The most important element of adaptation is to have an exceptionally strong organizational culture so that everyone from the top down knows—without ambiguity—what the organization's true values and principles are. People will be attracted to such a strong corporate culture, and anything can be accomplished.

In *Intangibles: The Unexpected Traits of High-Performing Healthcare Leaders*, Dr. Amer Kaissi has consolidated results from a broad array of research data from multiple studies, as well as his own interviews, to provide readers with a refreshing level of learning.

As a healthcare leader for more than 45 years, with 31 as a CEO, I continue to be a student. What Dr. Kaissi shows is that regardless of your station in leadership, from student to CEO, you can learn from others about the significance of personal characteristics.

Healthcare is more complex and demanding than ever before. With new presidential leadership, the Affordable Care Act and many policies in our economy will be challenged and renegotiated. Leaders will have to be prepared to try new ideas, and innovation will take center stage. Competition will dominate organizational strategy, and information technology will create an ever more aggressive environment. Things are getting tough, but experience has proven to me that healthcare has never been easy. Aggressive negotiations with payers, suppliers, and physicians have challenged us, but the characteristics of humility, compassion, kindness, and generosity have proven to be lifesavers in all situations.

A career is not about success alone, as success is often fleeting. It is about significance. Do I exceed one's expectations and make a lasting difference rather than a temporary one? The characteristics that Dr. Kaissi shares in his book are proven ways to lead. They are the human side of the enterprise. How you treat others is a calling card that will elevate your performance beyond those who seek results by any means.

For students, young careerists, and seasoned veterans, *Intangibles* is an important read—not once, but many times.

Douglas D. Hawthorne, LFACHE
Founding Chief Executive Officer Emeritus,
Texas Health Resources

Preface

"OH NO—NOT ANOTHER leadership book!"

I know what you're thinking, because I've had the same thought myself, many times. Dismay is my typical reaction when I stumble across a new leadership-related title. Bookstores are saturated with such publications. Just venture to your public library and you'll find volume after volume promising readers that they too can become successful leaders if only they apply the book's advice and principles.

So why did I spend two years of my life adding to the stack of leadership books? Because I realized that among all the books that are available, there was a significant void, especially in healthcare. While there are many excellent texts with great advice, most of them were written by previous or current executives who aim to distill the lessons they have learned over their careers into a number of principles or recommendations. However, with all due respect to these authors, one person's experience, no matter how rich and significant, is just that—*one* person's experience.

What's lacking in leadership books, especially in healthcare, is evidence-based practices: practices that have been proven to be effective by a large number of people, in a variety of different settings, over time. Evidence is what I attempt to provide in this book; I combed through many studies, sources, and expert wisdom to uncover the truth. As a healthcare administration professor, I spend a lot of time interacting with students and graduates working in hospitals and other healthcare organizations. Observing the careers of some 600 emerging leaders over the past 15 years has given me good insight into leadership styles. Moreover, I interviewed 20 current and retired healthcare leaders, providers, and experts on leadership-related issues and collected data from more than 500 employees, supervisors, middle managers, and executives in nine health systems.

If you're hoping that, by reading this book, you'll get the five principles of management, the seven habits of success, or the nine rules of leadership, then you'll be disappointed. Also, there are no made-up buzzwords and no terms that are copyrighted with a little © next to them. This book isn't self-help either—another how-to guide to becoming a better person or a more effective boss.

What you *will* see in this book are findings from other studies and results from my own research data. You'll also find insights from people I've interviewed and from interviews reported by others. For example, you'll learn how the philosophy of a nursing student relates to compassion in leadership. You'll distill leadership lessons from a nun (turned CEO), a highly successful Scottish soccer coach, a strong and caring vice president, and a retired executive who has a charter school named after him. You'll also uncover what it means to be an asshole at work, what the nice guy syndrome is all about, and how the *Divergent* book series is biased against nice people.

I decided to write this book in part because I believe, as do many others, that we have a significant problem in our country today. In a recent report published by the Harvard Graduate School of Education, 10,000 middle and high school students from 33 schools across the nation were surveyed. The students were asked to rank what's most important to them: achieving at a high level, happiness (feeling good most of the time), or caring for others. The majority of the respondents (48 percent) picked achievement, 30 percent picked happiness, and only 22 percent picked caring as their top priority. As one respondent noted, "If you are not happy, life is nothing. After that, you want to do well. And after that, expend any excess energy on others" (Making Caring Common Project 2014, 1).

These findings expose a serious gap between what parents and teachers describe as their priorities for students and what the students perceive as adults' priorities. Almost all parents say that they're deeply invested in raising caring, ethical children and that they see these moral qualities as more important than achievement. Data from teacher surveys suggest that teachers also view preparing youth to be caring as more important than preparing them for achievement. The young, however, appear to be hearing a different message. When asked about the priorities of their parents and teachers, most young people in the survey said that the adults in their lives are more concerned about achievement than caring. Despite what they say, many parents and teachers are prioritizing grades and results over children's compassion and kindness toward others.

Other research examining narcissism and empathy among college students has shown that the majority of current students score higher on narcissism and lower on empathy today than their counterparts did 30 years ago (Twenge and Foster 2010; Konrath, O'Brien, and Hsing 2011). This shift is especially important for me as an educator because these are the same young people I encounter every day in the classroom and send off every year to leadership positions. If these results apply to graduate healthcare administration students (and there's no reason to believe that they wouldn't), then only one in five emerging healthcare leaders believes that caring for others is a top priority. This figure implies that our healthcare system, and society in general, have some serious challenges. The real issue isn't just that youths prioritize achievement and happiness over caring—it's that they see these priorities as mutually exclusive. In their minds, it's not possible to be successful *and* caring. They believe that being compassionate and kind to others might deter them from advancing in their careers.

Therefore, this book is an exploration of what great minds, philosophers, researchers, and healthcare executives have to say about the role of humility, compassion, kindness, and generosity in leadership. At the heart of the book is a simple question: Can leaders embody these characteristics and be successful at the same time? As I explore this issue, other important questions will emerge, which I'll tackle in part 2. For example, with all the changes in the healthcare sector, what kind of traits will future healthcare leaders need? Can leaders balance humility, compassion, kindness, and generosity with having a strong personality? With getting things done? With producing results? Is being compassionate and kind viewed by some as going soft, as diluting hard decisions and watering down a solid focus on outcomes? Is humility viewed as being weak? What are the advantages of being compassionate, kind, generous, and humble? Are leaders who possess these traits better at inspiring others and guiding their organizations toward success? After addressing these core questions, I'll turn my attention in part 3 to issues of gender, age, and training. How do men and women differ in their perceptions of humility, compassion, kindness, and generosity? Are there generational differences in how leadership is perceived? Finally, are these traits inborn, or can they be learned through training and practice?

I won't get too hung up on definitions. When conducting academic studies to be published in peer-reviewed journals, researchers typically go to great lengths to disentangle specific concepts from each other. But for the sake of simplicity, I'll take the essentials of that research and present it in an easy-to-understand way, without spending too much time on the etiological and conceptual differences between humility, compassion, kindness, and generosity, and their close cousins: empathy, niceness, altruism, and graciousness.

Some of you may be starting to roll your eyes and think that this all sounds New Agey. "I don't have time for humility and kindness," you say, "I have a budget to meet," "I have a deal to close," or "I have a promotion to get." I understand your reaction. I'm not, by nature, a touchy-feely person. In fact, many people who know me were caught by surprise when I told them that I was writing a book about humility and compassion. Most of my colleagues, students, family members, and friends would describe me as pragmatic. This point is important—you don't have to be some New Age seeker of happiness to appreciate the importance of how you present yourself and how you treat others. The evidence that I'll present suggests that the more concerned you are about cold, hard metrics and objective performance outcomes, the more attention you should pay to humility and compassion.

Others may be thinking of humility as a no-brainer. "Of course I want to be humble and compassionate. Who doesn't want to treat others well?" I can tell you that the value of humility is not straightforward, especially early in your career when you're competing for limited opportunities for recognition, promotion, and advancement. When you're trying to make a name for yourself and stand out from the pack, acting with humility and treating others with compassion and kindness may not be among your top priorities.

The healthcare field is becoming increasingly competitive, especially after the passage of the Affordable Care Act in 2010 and its attempted repeal by the Trump administration in 2017. Leaders of hospitals and health systems have to negotiate hard with physicians, payers, competitors, governing boards, and other health systems. In this cutthroat environment, "tough" leadership traits such as aggressiveness, competitiveness, and mercilessness may seem more useful than "soft" traits such as humility, compassion, kindness, and generosity.

But evidence emerging from different fields shows that as things get tougher, humble leaders who serve, care, and treat others with compassion and kindness are very successful in achieving results for their organizations and their communities in the long run. These leaders aren't weak. They're humble and kind, but they're also ambitious and strong-willed—leaders who hold themselves and others accountable through clear expectations. When you add humble to ambitious, you get *humbitious*. (Okay, I admit—this is a made-up word.) I believe that humbitious leaders are the high-performing healthcare leaders of the future.

The idea for writing this book emerged in the fall of 2014 while I was on sabbatical. But in fact, its seeds have been germinating all my life. The leadership style that I advocate is one that my parents have always espoused: They're humble, compassionate, kind, and generous, but they also set clear expectations and explain consequences. My father is the kindest person I know, but no one ever viewed him as weak. My mother is the strongest person I know, but she was never perceived as intimidating. Together, they combined humility and ambition, kindness and strength. While they were both leaders in their respective jobs (my father was a bank executive, my mother was the director of a nonprofit), they best demonstrated their approach at home. They treated my brother and me with care and love, but they set clear expectations about good behavior and good grades. When we messed up, we knew there would consequences. I aspire to use this parenting style with my own children, and I also believe it is applicable to leadership relations today, especially in healthcare.

This book is written for you: the undergraduate and graduate students, the early careerists and the emerging leaders in healthcare. My plan is to reach you before you're set in your ways. I won't be giving you any prescriptive answers, but my hope is that, as you turn these pages, you'll begin to ask yourself some profound questions about caring, leadership styles, and behaviors. I hope to push you to start making some changes in how you behave with others as a leader and how you treat the people who will be working with you and for you. I hope that you'll start working toward becoming a humbitious leader. That's why this is a different type of leadership book that will be worth your time.

Amer Kaissi, PhD
Trinity University

REFERENCES

Konrath, S. H., E. H. O'Brien, and C. Hsing. 2011. "Changes in Dispositional Empathy in American College Students over Time: A Meta-analysis." *Personality and Social Psychology Review* 15 (2): 180–98.

Making Caring Common Project. 2014. *The Children We Mean to Raise*. Harvard Graduate School of Education. Accessed April 6, 2017. http://mcc.gse.harvard.edu/files/gse-mcc/files/mcc-research-report.pdf.

Twenge, J. M., and J. D. Foster. 2010. "Birth Cohort Increases in Narcissistic Personality Traits Among American College Students, 1982–2009." *Social Psychological and Personality Science* 1 (1): 99–106.

Acknowledgments

I AM DEEPLY grateful to several individuals for their advice and help. Mrs. Laura Monroe graciously donated her time and expertise to assist with research and review, while expecting nothing in return. Without her vital help, this book wouldn't have been completed. Ms. Theresa Rothschadl, my editor at Health Administration Press, provided exceptional editorial attention that was supportive, humorous, and rigorous. Dr. James Begun at the University of Minnesota, always my mentor and adviser, offered valuable advice when I first embarked on this project. Mr. John Hornbeak and Dr. Jody Rogers from Trinity University provided highly appreciated advice and encouragement. Dr. Deneese Jones, vice president of academic affairs at Trinity University, offered strongly encouraging words of support about the importance of this topic. Several executives were very accommodating and gave me permission to collect survey data from their organizations: Mr. Derrick Cuenca, Mrs. Sally Hurt-Deitch, Mr. Craig Desmond, Mr. Dale Flowers, Mr. Enrique Gallegos, Mr. Javier Irruegas, Mr. Bruce Lawrence, and Mr. Marc Strode. Twenty leaders and experts (listed in the appendix) graciously agreed to be interviewed and to share their expertise and time. Professor Edward Schumacher, chair of the Department of Health Care Administration at Trinity University, was very supportive and understanding in accommodating the time demands this project made. Graduate research assistant Dillon Rai provided important research support. Finally, I am always indebted to the countless blessings of the Almighty God for the accomplishment of this and all other projects in my life.

PART 1

Introduction

CHAPTER 1

Leadership Intangibles

1

ON A WARM day in July 2004, Rebecca Ivatury, a nursing student at the University of Central Florida, sat down to contemplate her nursing philosophy. Articulating a philosophy is common practice among nurses, and it can help young students clarify their values and reflect on how their beliefs fit with their professional practice. Rebecca had been thinking about hers for a while. After much self-reflection, she finally wrote:

> I believe that the patient should be treated as a whole human being. My first obligation is safety in caring for the patient. This obligation resides in providing proficient care that will benefit the patient. As a competent nurse, I will apply what I have learned from theory and implement care that is based on research that benefits the patient. My next obligation resides in treating the human spirit of the patient, by this I mean providing empathy and compassion for the patient as a fellow human being. I know that my job satisfaction will occur when I have made the best possible choices in the care of my patient as a whole human being. (Ivatury 2016)

Rebecca loved being a nurse, and she enjoyed taking care of patients. Even when they asked the same questions over and over and when they pushed the call button many times, they never bothered her. At the end of each day, she always felt fulfilled because she had helped them feel better.

Judging from the numerous cards and notes that she has received over the years, patients really appreciated what she did for them. One day, for example, a previous patient came back to see her after his hospital stay. He brought his granddaughter with him, and he gave Rebecca a thank-you note and a $50 restaurant gift card. He told Rebecca that when he was in the hospital, she once sat down with him and kindly explained to him how smoking was hurting his lungs. "I quit smoking and I never went back so I can be there for my granddaughter. I couldn't have done that without your help," he told her while fighting back his tears (Ivatury 2016).

Like millions of other healthcare professionals, Rebecca knew that compassion and kindness were a pivotal part of her job. The majority of nurses, doctors, and other direct care providers go into healthcare because they want to help others and exercise compassion and kindness. But does the same hold true for healthcare administrators in leadership positions? For nondirect care providers working in management and executive teams, are these traits a requirement? This book will explore the idea that leaders in healthcare administration are more effective at producing results and getting things done when they have what I call the *leadership intangibles*: humility, compassion, kindness, and generosity.

2

The idea that leaders can be humble and achieve great things isn't a new one. If we look back to ancient history, we find some fascinating examples. Cyrus the Great was the founder of the world's first empire and, by all accounts, a towering figure in the history of humankind. He is said to have built the Persian empire through kindness and care. "More important than the territory Cyrus conquered were his policies of tolerance and inclusion. . . . Cyrus recognized individual differences and appreciated what diversity could bring to his empire. He tried to win over his enemies through trust and inclusion—an approach that must have seemed amazing at a time when the usual tools of conquest were destruction, massacre, and enslavement," write Steve Forbes and John Prevas (2009, 44). Their noted book, *Power, Ambition, Glory*, explores the traits of great leaders of the ancient world and compares them to those of some contemporary business leaders.

Augustus, the great Roman emperor, was another humble historical leader. After the assassination of his great-uncle and adoptive father Julius Caesar, Augustus led Rome's transformation from republic to empire by combining military might, institution building, and lawmaking. Eventually he became Rome's sole ruler, laying the foundation for one of the most successful empires in history. Augustus was known for his personal humility, referring to himself as no more than Rome's *primus inter paris*, or "first among equals." Despite being the undisputed leader of millions and the richest man in the ancient world, he kept his ego in check and listened to others (Forbes and Prevas 2009).

3

Let's turn our attention back to the workplace. Many people will most likely recall an arrogant, abusive leader much more easily than a humble, compassionate one. We often refer to these leaders as "jerks" or "bullies." Robert Sutton, a professor of management science and engineering at Stanford University, irreverently calls them assholes! In 2003, he used the term *asshole at work* in an article that appeared in the prestigious *Harvard Business Review*. Sutton admits that he considered using more proper terms such as *jerk* or *bully* but felt that they were watered down and censored variations that "simply did not have the same ring of authenticity or emotional appeal" (2007, 3). After the article received widespread attention, he wrote a book addressing the same topic by the title of *The No Asshole Rule*.

According to Sutton, there are ways to spot an asshole. First, after talking to him, the other person feels oppressed, humiliated, de-energized, and belittled. Second, an asshole typically aims his venom at people who are less powerful than himself. On any given day, he may use personal insults, invade others' personal territory, initiate uninvited physical contact, and use verbal and nonverbal threats and intimidation. He also may insult others using sarcastic jokes and teasing, write withering e-mail flames, engage in public shaming or status degradation rituals, rudely interrupt others, use two-faced attacks, spray dirty looks, and treat others as if they're invisible (Sutton 2007). There are many negative effects of having assholes in the workplace, including reduced job satisfaction and productivity and trouble concentrating at work, and their actions can lead to serious damage to others. Their actions can also cause mental and physical health problems such as difficulty sleeping, anxiety, feelings of worthlessness, chronic fatigue, irritability, anger, and depression. The people involved extend beyond the victims themselves to their coworkers, family members, or friends, who suffer from the ripple effects of the abuse.

But perhaps the most significant impact of jerks is on organizational performance. The costs of increased turnover, absenteeism, decreased commitment to work, distraction, and impaired individual performance are well documented in psychological studies. The Total Cost of Assholes or TCA (yes, someone made that up and took the time to measure it!) at one company was estimated to be about $160,000 per salesperson in terms of time spent by management to monitor, contain, and discipline assholes; turnover; overtime cost; anger management; and training, among other costs (Sutton 2007).

Unpleasant people are a problem at any level but are especially harmful when they're in leadership positions. When people rise into positions of power, they tend to start acting in an abrasive way. They talk more, take what they want for themselves, disregard what other people say, ignore how their behavior affects others, and generally treat everyone with disdain and rudeness. It is human nature to act in this way with even small and insignificant power advantages. Imagine this experiment: A number of college students were divided into groups of three and were asked to discuss a long list of social issues (e.g., abortion, pollution). The researchers assigned one member of the group, at random, to be the leader who evaluated the recommendations of the other two. After 30 minutes, a plate of five cookies was brought to each group. The students who were assigned the power position were more likely to take a second cookie, chew with their mouths open, and get crumbs on their faces and on the table—all self-centered behaviors. So even in a short experiment, human beings become full of themselves as soon as they're given any type of power over others (Sutton 2007).

Given how dangerous assholes can be, why are they tolerated in our organizations and culture? Sutton maintains that the unspoken standard in American business, medicine, sports, and academia is that "the more often you are right and the more often you win, the bigger a jerk you can be" (Sutton 2007, 55). If we're honest, we have to admit that there are some advantages to being a jerk. Acting that way can sometimes makes you seem smarter than others and may help you obtain benefits at work. In an article titled "Brilliant But Cruel," Professor Teresa Amabile studied people's perception of positive and negative book reviews. She reports that people perceived negative reviewers as "more intelligent, competent, and expert than positive reviewers, even when the content of the positive review was independently judged as being of higher quality and greater forcefulness" (Amabile 1983, 146).

Many think that jerks are smarter or better than nice people. Reality television is full of examples that confirm Sutton's point: Simon Cowell on *American Idol*, Piers Morgan on *America's Got Talent*, and more recently, Kevin O'Leary (the ironically self-nicknamed "Mr. Wonderful") on *Shark Tank*. When these judges make demeaning comments and poke fun at contestants, most people automatically assume that they must be really good at what they do. While we may be fascinated by jerks on television, however, very few of us would want to work for them in real life.

A few years ago, like millions of people around the world, I rushed to the bookstore to get my hands on Walter Isaacson's biography of Steve Jobs. Like many others, I was mesmerized by the genius of Jobs, who almost single-handedly transformed personal computers, phones, mobile computers, music, and animation, and in the process, changed our lives forever.

As I dug deeper into Jobs's life and career, however, I gradually became troubled by his behavior and poor treatment of others. Isaacson presented evidence that Jobs was a tyrant who threw frequent tantrums and regularly yelled at his employees. In meetings, it was a common occurrence for him to say, "You asshole, you never do anything right" (Isaacson 2011, 124). As I understood the extent of Jobs's abuse, I started asking myself, Would he have been more successful if he had had better self-control and treated others in a more compassionate and kind way? Or would he have lost his mojo, so to speak, and become less successful? Six months after Jobs's death, Isaacson addressed some of these concerns in an article about leadership style: "When I pressed him [Jobs] on whether he could have gotten the same results while being nicer, he said perhaps so. 'But it's not who I am,' he said. 'Maybe there's a better way—a gentlemen's club where we all wear ties and speak in this Brahmin language and velvet code words—but I don't know that way, because I am middle-class from California'" (Isaacson 2012, 99).

How do we make sense of Jobs's example? I believe that Steve Jobs is the exception, rather than the rule. His behavior was tolerated, and many were loyal to him because they saw his passion for what he did, as well as his intelligence, creativity, and perfectionism. But that does not give the rest of us a license to abuse and mistreat others. This fact is of special importance for the many young people who consider Jobs a role model, especially those who think to themselves, "If Steve Jobs was a jerk and he was one of the most successful leaders in one of the most successful companies in the world, if I act like him, maybe I'll be successful too" (Williams 2015). Just because Steve Jobs abused people and was outrageously successful doesn't mean that other hopefuls can act the same way.

Another way to look at this issue is to admit that some intimidation and toughness can be beneficial in the workplace, especially when difficult changes are needed and people aren't ready to embrace them. Roderick Kramer, an experimental social psychologist and professor of organizational behavior at Stanford, calls Steve Jobs–type leaders the "great intimidators" (Kramer 2006, 2). These are the leaders who don't shy away from conflict and confrontation. Kramer suggests that a list of great intimidators would read a bit like a business leadership hall of fame: Sandy Weill, Rupert Murdoch, Andy Grove, Carly Fiorina, Larry Ellison, and Steve Jobs.

But the great intimidators, according to Kramer, aren't bullies who humiliate others to make themselves look good. Rather than being driven by their egos, these leaders are driven by vision. They're motivated to remove any obstacles, including human ones, that may stand in their way. The secret to their success is their political intelligence, which allows them to enact changes in the face of resistance and inertia (Kramer 2006). They appreciate the power of fear and anxiety, unashamedly leverage other people's weaknesses and insecurities, and use intimidation and hard power to exploit the anxieties they detect. Such leaders are able to intimidate and vanquish their rivals, bring clueless and lazy people to their senses, and motivate fear-driven performance and perfectionism. It isn't pretty, Kramer argues, but it works.

5

Michael C. Zucker is the former senior vice president and chief development officer at Baptist Health System in San Antonio, Texas, where he oversaw strategy, growth, and development for seven years. He has served in senior leadership roles with many healthcare organizations in a successful career spanning more than 25 years. Recently, he left Baptist Health System and cofounded Ranger Health.

I've known Mike for a while, and we regularly get together to catch up. When I was doing research for this book, I met with him for lunch at his favorite restaurant in San Antonio. When I explained to him what I was working on, he was intrigued by the topic and quick to offer his personal observations.

> My leadership style is very direct, perhaps similar to the well-known leadership styles of Jack Welch or Steve Jobs. I have witnessed an increasing trend among leaders in all levels who are not held accountable for their performance. I have experienced leaders that would rather not address the issues of weak performance at the expense of improving the organization's performance. These managers and leaders prefer to take the easier road of not addressing individual performance, perhaps due to someone being very tenured or well liked, or because they have no one to immediately backfill a leadership void that would be created. Regardless, this is a disservice to the organization, its employees, and customers. I would characterize this leadership style as leading by emotion. Having a balance of emotion and compassion in one's leadership style are certainly good characteristics, but not at the expense of accountability. In our industry, some leaders have placed so much emphasis on leading with compassion that it has come at the expense of being able to drive change quickly. (Zucker 2014)

Mike's leadership style can be characterized as direct and results oriented. Those who have worked with him say that he's not big on small talk and that he expects preparation and performance.

Mike rightly points out that this issue isn't either/or—that there is a continuum of compassion and kindness along which people

operate. For example, Mike has served for many years as a preceptor for healthcare administration graduate students. He describes
his approach with young residents as caring but not compassionate.
"My style with the students is one of 'hard love.' I don't shower the
administrative residents with constant and positive affirmation. I
will acknowledge a job well done when it is earned. Likewise, I will
spend 30 minutes with them after a meeting to discuss the learning
opportunities. I also expect few mistakes, well-written reports, and
quality work products, because we are making decisions based on
the residents' work. I truly care about their education and professional growth and will challenge them to perform, as it is part of
the learning experience" (Zucker 2014).

Hurley Smith is one of Mike's previous administrative residents,
having worked with him for a whole year on strategic and financial
projects. During that time, Hurley was given access to all meetings
and was allowed to get involved in a variety of different groups and
committees. Mike didn't hold Hurley's hand, and he rarely praised
him for doing what was expected. But Hurley recalls one special day:

> One afternoon, I was working on my desk outside of Mike's
> office and the top button on my jacket fell off, just before
> a big presentation. Panicked, I tried to stitch the button
> back. Mike saw me struggling with the string and needle.
> He came over and asked, "What the heck are you doing?"
> I explained the situation to him. He inquired, "How long
> have you had this jacket?" I told him that I've had it since
> high school. I was a poor graduate student at the time; I
> didn't have a large wardrobe. He said, "Hurley, you have
> outgrown this jacket. You can't wear this to the meeting
> today." So I went to the meeting and did the presentation
> without the jacket.
>
> After the meeting, Mike asked me to go have a drink
> with him. Once at the bar, he didn't waste any time on
> small talk, he went straight to business—it was so hard
> to hear. He said that I was spending way too much time

working on my computer at my desk and not enough time going out and learning things in the hospitals. That was one of the most intense, true coaching sessions in my life. Afterwards, he took me across the street to Jos. A. Bank and bought me a suit for $350. He said: "Now you look like you mean business." That is when I realized that, in his own way, Mike really cared about me. I will never forget that. (Smith 2016)

6

I hope that by now you're starting to realize that the issue of leader behavior and its effect on performance isn't as black and white as some might portray it. You can be compassionate and kind and also be a high performer. You can be intimidating and rude and be very successful. You can also be nice and caring and get nothing done, just as you can be a jerk and drive your organization into the ground. Like any other important aspect of leadership, there are no easy answers. There are no step-by-step manuals that you can follow to be more successful. As cliché as it might sound, *it depends*. It depends on your personality, your upbringing, the type of people you're leading, the kind of organization you work in, and the situation you're facing, among many other factors.

For instance, there is evidence that one's leadership style isn't stable over time, but rather varies from day to day. In other words, the same leader can be abusive one day and kind another. Leaders who often act like jerks may still have days in which they're compassionate and kind, and leaders who are humble and caring may have days in which they hurl insults at others (Barnes et al. 2015).

Evidence also exists that different leadership styles may be more effective depending on the followers' personal traits. For example, people who are high on agreeableness are generally courteous to others, prefer cooperation over competition, and are typically thoughtful and considerate. On the other hand, those low on agreeableness tend to get into arguments, are often skeptical of others' intentions, and are cynical and confrontational. In a recent study of college students in the Netherlands, participants worked collaboratively on a simulation exercise. After they finished the task, they received feedback on how they could have improved their performance from a team leader (an actor) via video streaming. In the first instance, the leader looked cheerful, spoke with an enthusiastic and upbeat tone of voice, and smiled frequently. In the second instance, the leader frowned a lot, spoke with an angry and irritable tone of voice, clenched his fists, and looked stern. The same message was delivered in both cases, with the leader expressing either happiness or anger though his facial expressions, vocal intonation, and bodily postures. The study results showed that followers who scored low on agreeableness performed better when the leader expressed anger rather than happiness. In contrast, highly agreeable followers performed better when the leader was cheerful and energetic. This result suggests that effective leaders can match their leadership style and emotional expressions to those of their followers (Van Kleef et al. 2010).

Also important to note is that a certain leadership style may work well in one situation but backfire in another. When the organization is facing highly volatile and risky conditions, a loud and rambunctious leader may do better than a humble consensus builder. "If we think of leadership styles as running along a continuum from very humble to dangerously brash and overconfident, it might be that different kinds of leadership styles operate better in some business environments than in others," notes John Banja, a medical ethicist at Emory University (Banja 2015, 52). Some historians view Winston Churchill's brash and sometimes arrogant style, for example, as one of the main reasons behind the Allied victory in World War II. However, immediately after the war ended, that style was less appreciated, and Churchill and his party were voted out of office.

Another factor of success rarely addressed in leadership books and studies is pure luck. Humble leaders attribute most of their achievements to external factors such as others' contributions, good fortune, and serendipity. John Hornbeak, the retired CEO of Methodist Health System in San Antonio, is one of those leaders who are always hesitant to take credit for organizational successes. He notes that "luck is understudied in leadership. Sometimes, we're successful because we are in the right place at the right time. And other times, we are successful because the competition screwed up, or one of their high-admitting doctors just fell into our lap" (Hornbeak 2014).

7

The studies and opinions highlighted in the previous sections suggest that context and luck can play an important role in affecting leadership effectiveness. But overall, the evidence shows that in most situations and in most organizations, the leadership intangibles of humility, compassion, kindness, and generosity can help leaders achieve more than intimidation and fear in the long run. In workplaces with cultures based on compassion rather than fear, talented individuals share their ideas more freely and dysfunctional internal competition is reduced. As a result, people tend to stick around, and turnover cost is lower.

The notion that a leader's style can become a long-term competitive advantage for her individual employees, team, and organization is one that Heidi Pandya strongly believes in. Heidi obtained her master's degree in healthcare administration in 2005 and went on to have a successful career in the competitive field of management consulting. Her style is "big on communicating, on interpersonal skills with my team and my clients." She wants others to enjoy coming to work and being around her, which makes them comfortable admitting their mistakes and talking about their problems with her. "They know that when they tell me about a problem, my first reaction is to understand and to find a solution, not to get frustrated or angry at them," she explains. While that style is compatible with Heidi's personality, it also allows her to achieve results in the long run. "I do that because this is who I am, but also because I want to build a team and retain people, I don't want to keep losing people and rehiring new ones and training them," she says (Pandya 2016).

Heidi has been a preceptor and mentor for many young residents and interns at a large global professional services firm. Despite her young age, they endearingly call her their "mother." Marisa Stansberry, one of the young consultants who were mentored by Heidi, explains how Heidi treated her:

> I always appreciated that Heidi would call me and check in on me, even when I wasn't staffed on a project with her. She always asked me what she could do to help me. I would obviously have never taken her up on that, because no matter how swamped I was, I knew she had it worse, but it meant the world to me that she would ask. She never made me feel like she is too important or high up the food chain to roll her sleeves up and work, and that made me want to work even harder for her.

Heidi led her team by example by holding herself to high standards and getting things done on time. When the team achieved its goals, she always gave them credit: "If we had to work until 3am to get something done for a partner, she mentioned us by name to that partner the next day to give us credit. On group calls, she always said all the credit goes to her team and remembered what each one of us contributed specifically to the project" (Stansberry 2016).

When leaders behave in positive ways, good things happen in organizations. In a study of 800 employees in 18 organizations across different sectors, scholars Kim Cameron, David Bright, and Arran Caza (2004) found that recently downsized organizations did better when their leaders were virtuous. Virtuousness means that leaders acted with kindness, compassion, forgiveness, and gratitude. This finding is especially important because after downsizing, employees typically have negative perceptions of their organizations. These perceptions, demonstrated by grudge holding, hostility, and retribution seeking, can often lead to performance deterioration. But when leaders are virtuous, the organization is able to keep its employees and maintain its innovation and profitability. Cameron uses the term *positive leadership*, which he describes as promoting virtuous behaviors and allowing people to thrive at work while insisting on strict performance standards (Cameron 2012, x).

8

Sir Alex Ferguson is the most successful coach in the history of British soccer, if not all of international soccer. Between 1986 and 2013, he guided his team, Manchester United, to no fewer than 38 local and international trophies. He was knighted by the queen of England in 1999 for his role in guiding his team to a historic *treble* (winning the English League, the English Cup, and the European Champions League in one season), an unprecedented feat at the time. He had the ability to combine youthful players with experienced players, build a winning team, and restart the process every five to six years, when the team would reach the end of its performance cycle (BBC News 1999).

Any casual fan would describe Ferguson as a fierce, ruthless coach who stopped at nothing in order to win. When his players underperformed, he gave them the infamous "hairdryer" treatment at halftime: He would single out one or two players who made a mistake or played particularly poorly, standing directly in front of them in the middle of the locker room. He would shout and scream in their faces for 10 to 15 minutes, often questioning whether they deserved to play for Manchester United. When he noticed that a player's form had dipped because of injury or age, or that a player was questioning his authority in public, he ruthlessly cut them from the club altogether (Sportsmail Daily Reporter 2012).

His relationship with reporters wasn't any friendlier. When the BBC aired a documentary in 2004 that made allegations about Ferguson's son, he imposed a seven-year ban on all BBC reporters, refusing to talk to them or to appear on any BBC program.

Ferguson also spared no criticism for rival coaches. For example, he had an especially tense relationship with the French manager of Arsenal, Arsene Wenger. After an especially fierce Manchester United–Arsenal battle that ended with a player for the rival team throwing pizza at him in the tunnel after the game, Ferguson called Wenger a "disgrace" (*Guardian* 2011).

But underneath that famous tough-guy facade, Ferguson showed glimpses of compassion and kindness that took many people by surprise. Cristiano Ronaldo, one of the best players in the world and a current icon of the game, was recruited by Ferguson to play for Manchester United when he was only 18 years old. He often talks about the special bond that he had with Ferguson. One day, before an especially important game, Ronaldo's father fell sick. So Ronaldo went to talk to Ferguson. He described (in his then-broken English) what happened:

> When my daddy was sick in London, and he was in hospital very bad in a coma, I had a conversation with him [Ferguson] and I said: "Boss, I don't feel good." We are in a key moment in the Champions League, and I said I don't feel good and I wanna see my dad. He said: "Cristiano—you wanna go one day, two days, one week? You can go. I'm going to miss you here because you are important, but your daddy is the [priority]." When he told me that, I feel like this guy is unbelievable. He the father of football for me. (Parthasarathi 2008)

Given Ronaldo's immense talent and his importance to the team, it would have been understandable if Ferguson had insisted that he stay with the team and play. Instead, he demonstrated great compassion by allowing the young superstar to be with his family.

Ferguson's compassion didn't just apply to his best players, on whom he depended for success. Many describe the special bond that he had with the "little people" at Manchester United: those who did the laundry, maintained the lawn, or worked in the cafeteria.

Ferguson paid special attention to them, going out of his way to show his appreciation for their work. For him, these were the unsung heroes of Manchester United, who often stayed at the club longer than anyone else. Most of them took the bus to come serve the super-rich players who paraded to the training grounds in their Porsches and Ferraris. Given his humble origins growing up as the son of a shipbuilder in the impoverished town of Govan in Scotland, it was easy for Ferguson to feel an affinity with those individuals. He believes that "kindness is a universal language regardless of age, nationality, or religion" (Ferguson 2011).

In his recent book *Leading*, Ferguson explains the secret to his long-standing success: "You don't get the best out of people by hitting them with an iron rod. You do so by gaining their respect, getting them accustomed to triumphs, and convincing them that they are capable of improving their performance. I cannot think of any manager who succeeded for any length of time by presiding over a reign of terror. It turns out that the two most powerful words in the English language are 'well done.' Much of leadership is about extracting that extra 5 percent of performance that individuals did not know they possessed" (Ferguson and Moritz 2015, 118). After retiring from coaching in 2013, Ferguson has been teaching a leadership course at Harvard Business School, explaining how he combined compassion and ruthlessness to lead his high-performing teams to numerous successes over the years.

9

Let's circle back to Rebecca, the nurse. After working for ten years in nursing, she went back to school to get a master's degree in healthcare administration. A few years after she graduated, I asked her to think back about her nursing philosophy and how it relates to her new role in administration. She noted, "What my nursing philosophy meant is that a nurse has to have compassion and kindness, but that is not enough by itself. It should be coupled with competency and technical skills. You can't have a compassionate nurse that doesn't know how to start an IV or can't make accurate clinical decisions. The same applies for leaders—they have to be nice, but they also have to hold people to a standard. You care about your people but you don't want to be seen as lenient. The successful leader has to be kind and respected" (Ivatury 2016). The bedrock argument of this book is the following: Effective leaders are admired for their humility, compassion, kindness, and generosity and are respected for their ambition, toughness, determination, and competence. They're *humbitious.*

REFERENCES

Amabile, T. M. 1983. "Brilliant But Cruel: Perceptions of Negative Evaluators." *Journal of Experimental Social Psychology* 19 (2): 146–56.

Banja, J. 2015. "Humility and Leadership: Can Healthcare Organizations Benefit from the Traits of Humble Leaders?" *Healthcare Executive*, January/February, 50–53.

Barnes, M. C., L. Lucianetti, P. D. Bhave, and S. M. Christian. 2015. "'You Wouldn't Like Me When I'm Sleepy': Leaders' Sleep, Daily Abusive Supervision, and Work Unit Engagement." *Academy of Management Journal* 58 (5): 1419–37.

BBC News. 1999. "Knighthood for Treble-Winner Ferguson." Published June 12. http://news.bbc.co.uk/2/hi/special _report/1999/06/99/queens_birthday_honours/366908.stm.

Cameron, K. 2012. *Positive Leadership: Strategies for Extraordinary Performance.* San Francisco: Berrett-Koehler Publishers.

Cameron, K., D. Bright, and A. Caza. 2004. "Exploring the Relationships Between Organizational Virtuousness and Performance." *American Behavioral Scientist* 47 (6): 766–90.

Ferguson, A. 2011. "Letter to David Jamily." Written September 28. http://kindnessuk.com/kind_quotes.php.

Ferguson, A., and M. Moritz. 2015. *Leading: Learning from Life and My Years at Manchester United*. New York: Hachette Books.

Forbes, S., and J. Prevas. 2009. *Power, Ambition, Glory: The Stunning Parallels Between Great Leaders of the Ancient World and Today . . . and the Lessons You Can Learn*. New York: Crown Publishing Group.

Guardian. 2011. "Sir Alex Ferguson Lifts Seven-Year Ban on Talking to BBC." Published August 25. www.theguardian.com /media/2011/aug/25/alex-ferguson-lifts-bbc-ban.

Hornbeak, J. 2014. Personal interview. September 12.

Isaacson, W. 2012. "The Real Leadership Lessons of Steve Jobs." *Harvard Business Review*. Published April. https://hbr .org/2012/04/the-real-leadership-lessons-of-steve-jobs.

———. 2011. *Steve Jobs*. New York: Simon & Schuster.

Ivatury, R. 2016. Phone interview. February 1.

Kramer, R. M. 2006. "The Great Intimidators." *Harvard Business Review*. Published February. https://hbr.org/2006/02 /the-great-intimidators.

Pandya, H. 2016. Personal interview. September 16.

Parthasarathi, S. 2008. "Arsene Wegner vs. Sir Alex Ferguson: An Intense Rivalry." *Bleacher Report*. Published September 14. http://bleacherreport.com/articles/57691-arsene-wenger-vs -sir-alex-ferguson-an-intense-rivalry.

Smith, H. 2016. Phone interview. February 12.

Sportsmail Daily Reporter. 2012. "There's Nothing Worse! Rooney Sheds Light on Ferguson's 'Hairdryer' Treatment as He Recalls Fiery Tirades." *Daily Mail*. Published September 14. www .dailymail.co.uk/sport/football/article-2203127/Wayne-Rooney -sheds-light-Sir-Alex-Fergusons-hairdryer.html.

Stansberry, M. 2016. E-mail correspondence with the author. December 21.

Sutton, R. 2007. *The No Asshole Rule.* New York: Hachette Book Group.

Van Kleef, G., A. C. Homan, B. Beersma, and D. van Knippenberg. 2010. "On Angry Leaders and Agreeable Followers: How Leaders' Emotions and Followers' Personalities Shape Motivation and Team Performance." *Psychological Science* 21 (12): 1827–34.

Williams, R. 2015. "Leaders: We Love Humble Leaders But Idolize Narcissists." *Psychology Today.* Published March 17. www.psychologytoday.com/blog/wired-success/201503 /leaders-we-love-humble-leaders-idolize-narcissists.

Zucker, M. 2014. Personal interview. November 19.

PART 2

Leadership Traits

CHAPTER 2

Humility

1

In 2014, Tony Hsieh, the cofounder and CEO of billion-dollar online empire Zappos, moved from his deluxe condo to a 240-square-foot trailer in downtown Las Vegas. Hsieh, who is estimated to be worth $780 million, could choose to live anywhere he wanted. But he decided to leave all luxury behind and to live an ordinary life because he wanted to be more in touch with his community and to have more experiences connecting with other people. "For me, experiences are more meaningful than stuff," he said after the move. "I have way more experiences here at [the trailer park]" (Totten 2015). To that end, he installed a community campfire and a shared kitchen for use with his neighbors. Every night at the trailer park, the residents gather round to talk, share ideas, and watch movies on a blow-up screen.

At Zappos, Hsieh doesn't operate out of the usual large corner office with plush furniture and an amazing view. Instead, he works from a desk in the middle of a sea of cubicles, just like everyone else. He's soft-spoken and deferential, and he makes his schedule available online for everyone inside and outside the company to see. He's the embodiment of the humbitious leader, a new breed of corporate leaders who are changing the way business is done.

But his humility isn't just about publicity stunts. It's also owning up to mistakes. In May of 2010, a pricing mistake on a Zappos sister site, 6pm.com, cost the company $1.6 million in revenue in just six short hours. The typical business reaction to this situation would be to find the culprit—someone in pricing—and fire that person. But at Zappos, Hsieh took to the Internet and explained to customers what really happened:

> We have a pricing engine that runs and sets prices according to the rules it is given by business owners. Unfortunately, the way to input new rules into the current version of our pricing engine requires near-programmer skills to manipulate, and a few symbols were missed in the coding of a new rule, which resulted in items that were sold exclusively on 6pm.com to have a maximum price of $49.95. . . . To those of you asking if anybody was fired, the answer is no, nobody was fired—this was a learning experience for all of us. Even though our terms and conditions state that we do not need to fulfill orders that are placed due to pricing mistakes, and even though this mistake cost us over $1.6 million, we felt that the right thing to do for our customers was to eat the loss and fulfill all the orders that had been placed before we discovered the problem. (Gelles 2015)

Despite the short-term losses, Zappos earned long-term credit with customers who appreciated the down-to-earth way it dealt with the problem.

Following Hsieh's example, employees at Zappos are allowed to take as much time as needed to interact with customers and solve their problems. When talking with people, they don't have a script—rather, they have the freedom to do whatever it takes to make things right for the customer. When new employees are hired, they spend two weeks in training, taking calls from customers. Later, they have the option of enrolling in a training program that allows them to develop additional skills. The training is optional, but the employees who complete the training receive a small pay increase. The employees are empowered to decide how they solve customer problems and when to take the additional training at their own pace. These policies, and many other activities at Zappos, allow the company to reach Hsieh's larger vision: "To deliver happiness to the world." Tony Hsieh's personal humility and the corresponding culture at Zappos is a breath of fresh air in a world that constantly rewards arrogance and narcissism. In the next section, we'll explore humility as a virtue and its recent applications in leadership.

2

The word *humility* comes from the Latin *humus*, which means "earth" (not to be confused with the delicious Middle Eastern dip). For the ancient Greeks, being humble was understood as being close to the earth or being low, which was not worthy of praise. For this reason, kings made subjects bow low before them. The thinkers of the time argued that a humble existence was, by definition, an abject one. You didn't *choose* to be humble, because the way you acted was determined by your status in society. If you had a noble birth, then acting with humility was considered shameful. Similarly, someone with modest lineage who strived for high status was considered foolish. While it's true that the Greeks didn't view humility as a virtue, they did caution against extremely high levels of pride. They coined the term *hubris*, or overconfidence, which they thought could blind a person and lead to his downfall.

One of the most influential works on humility comes to us from the thirteenth-century theologian Saint Thomas Aquinas, who studied it in the context of the Christian faith. He argues that being humble allowed man to properly subject himself to God, thus leading to detachment from self and to a healthy self-abasement (Aquinas 1917). Note that Aquinas doesn't see any contradiction between humility and greatness (which he called magnanimity). For him, those two traits complement one another because "a twofold virtue is necessary with regard to the difficult good: one, to temper and restrain the mind, lest it tend to high things immoderately; and this belongs to the virtue of humility: and another to strengthen the mind against despair, and urge it on to the pursuit of great things according to right reason; and this is magnanimity" (Aquinas 1917). This idea of combining humility and ambition, or what some call *humbition*, is an important one for our understanding of humility in leadership. Fast forward a few hundred years, and America's founding fathers were grappling with similar ideas. They recognized the importance of humility and desired to be humble, but they were also ambitious and wished to make their mark through the greatness of their actions (Bobb 2013).

Our longtime fascination with humility has been replaced with some mixed feelings in the present day. Most people want others around them to be humble, but they themselves behave with arrogance to receive attention and rewards. "Though the virtue of humility is occasionally praised in some faraway tribe, remote religious order, or politician's rural birthplace, the reality of our fame-addled and power hungry existence today means that arrogance is rewarded and humility is ignored," writes author and president of the Bill of Rights Institute David Bobb. "Ego trips are occasions for everyday media adulation," he adds (Bobb 2013, 4). Many people believe that the humble are shy wimps. Hard-charging individuals who want to succeed in business cannot imagine themselves sitting humbly on the sidelines. They feel the need to toot their own horns so that others notice them and feel impressed by their achievements.

3

Despite the abundance of arrogance in every arena of life, humility has recently made a surprise comeback as a sought-after virtue in business. For example, a recent article in the *Journal of Business Ethics* argues that "an excellent manager can and must be an ethical and, therefore, a humble manager. And this by no means implies any obstacle to her human and professional flourishing, her success within the firm or her reputation in society. In fact, quite the opposite: the humble leader is precisely the person who is best quali-fied to transform his firm into a profitable, successful, and respected organization" (Argandona 2015, 70).

The *Wall Street Journal* also recently reported that humility is becoming the flavor du jour among executives in large companies. After poor financial performance, Procter & Gamble's CEO, A. G. Lafley, faced the company's investors with a humble tone, shoul-dering the responsibility and assuring them that his successor will do better. Boards are also increasingly looking for humble leaders. When Krispy Kreme Doughnuts was looking for a CEO, its main requirement was a humble servant leader. The job went to Tony Thompson, who "exhibited those two characteristics strongly" (Lub-lin 2015). Similarly, humility is what Google is looking for in its new hires. "Your end goal is what can we do together to problem-solve. I've contributed my piece, and then I step back. [It's about] intellectual humility. Without humility, you are unable to learn," says Lazlo Bock, Google's senior vice president of people operations (Prime and Salib 2014b).

What does humble leadership actually mean? The five main foundations of humility as it applies to business include *fallibility*, *vulnerability*, *transparency*, *inadequacy*, and *interdependency* (Hoeks-tra, Bell, and Peterson 2008). A leader who accepts her own fallibility is one who admits to herself, "I make mistakes." This admission is different from the common view that mistakes happen in a random way. Rather, the leader admits that she, herself, messes up, and makes peace with the idea that followers don't expect her to be perfect. When the leader embraces fallibility, she is freed from living out the charade of perfectionism and the facade of never being wrong. This stage is followed by telling followers, "I need your patience," which allows the leader to demonstrate a level of authenticity that is appealing to them. Because everyone already knows that leaders make mistakes, hearing the leader admit to them is refreshing, which in turn creates an environment of authenticity in which everyone can openly admit to their own mistakes (Hoekstra, Bell, and Peter-son 2008). Nowhere is this atmosphere more important than in healthcare organizations, where a culture of openness and safety can help prevent medical mistakes and injuries.

It isn't enough for leaders to acknowledge that they generally make mistakes. They need to admit the specific situation in which they made a miscalculation, decided on a wrong option, or acted in a suboptimal way. Only when they do so and admit that they have contributed to the problem do leaders become vulnerable. This vulnerability comes in the form of confessing, "I was wrong." When a major crisis is under way, humble leaders look in the mirror and admit that their decisions and actions have contributed to that crisis. They look their employees in the eye and courageously say, "I need your forgiveness." This gesture generates reconciliation, which allows the leader and followers to move forward with a clean slate and no ill feelings (Hoekstra, Bell, and Peterson 2008).

As leaders climb the corporate ladder, their responsibilities increase and their jobs become more complex. Specific expertise in their areas of specialization becomes insufficient to deal with all aspects of the executive position. Humble leaders don't pretend that they know it all. Rather, when faced with unfamiliar situations or especially challenging circumstances, they bravely admit to their followers, "I don't know." Then they say, "I need your ideas." This request allows creative thinking and innovation to flow through the organization. When talented employees see their leader make that admission, their natural response is to bring forth their best ideas. Transparency encourages collaboration, which is necessary for dealing with complex issues and challenges (Hoekstra, Bell, and Peterson 2008).

Just as humble leaders admit that they don't know it all, they also realize that they can't do it all. They're aware of their own inadequacy and are willing to delegate important responsibilities to their subordinates. The humble leader admits to herself, "I can't do it all," then announces to her followers, "I need your talents." This admission allows her to prevent stress and burnout for herself, which is necessary for a healthy work–life balance. For the employees, the invitation to contribute their talent enables them to unleash their ideas and actions, which in turn provides them with the chance to reach their full potential (Hoekstra, Bell, and Peterson 2008).

Finally, humble leaders are other-centered rather than self-centered. They say to themselves, "I am not here for me." They recognize that their main purpose is to serve the organization and its people. This perception of the world enables them to view their employees as partners in the pursuit of organizational goals, which pushes them to announce, "I need your collaboration." This interdependency triggers the need to develop employees so they can improve and grow to achieve their own dreams, as well as to help reach organizational goals (Hoekstra, Bell, and Peterson 2008).

These five foundations of humble leadership are intertwined and interrelated. They come as a package—a truly humble leader can't have one and not the others. The results of humble leadership (authenticity, reconciliation, innovation, work–life balance, talent development) are the building blocks for a humble leader's journey toward high performance and toward leaving a legacy behind.

4

The thinking of leadership experts echoes the foundations of humble leadership. In his book *Leading at a Higher Level,* well-known author and management authority Ken Blanchard (2010, 275) states that "true leadership—the essence of what people long for and want desperately to follow—implies a certain humility that is appropriate and elicits the best response from people." He argues that the main obstacle preventing people from becoming effective leaders is their own ego, which he refers to as "**e**dging **g**ood **o**ut and putting yourself in the center."

Similarly, author and leadership consultant Bruna Martinuzzi argues that the best type of leaders are "Mensch leaders." *Mensch* is a Yiddish word that means a person of integrity and honor. Some of the characteristics of a Mensch are humility, empathy, and generosity. Martinuzzi views humility in leadership as maintaining pride in who we are—in our achievements and worth—without arrogance. She notes that Mensch leaders have an unassuming strength and a quiet confidence, without the urge to constantly sell themselves and their triumphs (Martinuzzi 2009).

In the notable book *Leading with Humility*, authors Rob Nielsen, Jennifer Marrone, and Holly Ferraro (2013) present a comprehensive approach to understanding humility in leadership. Humble leaders, they argue, are self-aware, open, low in self-focus, and other oriented, and they have a wide perspective. However, the authors suggest that humility isn't the same thing as modesty. Modest people underrepresent the importance of their positive traits and contributions and downplay the importance of their achievements. Humble people, on the other hand, don't hold themselves in low regard. Rather, they have a very good understanding of their own strengths and weaknesses, and they share them with others. Their main message isn't "I am weak" but rather "I have strengths and weaknesses." Most important, humble leaders don't display a reluctance to act. On the contrary, they believe that there is a vision beyond themselves worth moving toward. They make decisions that allow them to serve the collective interests and needs of others. They're very confident, but theirs is not the "I know I can do it—all of it—by myself, if I must" type of confidence. The confidence of humble leaders comes from the understanding that it isn't just about them—they believe in a vision that brings people together to accomplish a common purpose.

These opinions suggest that humility in leadership can lead to effectiveness and success. But what is the logic behind this assumption? First, humble leaders tend to share the credit for organizational accomplishments with others. Team members feel that they're being acknowledged and recognized for their contributions and as a result demonstrate strong satisfaction with their jobs. Their loyalty to the leader and to the organization increases over time, and voluntary turnover decreases. Because their efforts are being rewarded, they tend to expend more effort, thus resulting in better outcomes for themselves and for the organization.

Second, humble leaders give their followers a sense of ownership over work. Because they don't claim to know everything, they're willing to listen to suggestions and to give freedom to ideas. They specify the boundaries and clarify the expectations and end goals, but they let their team members feel as if they own the project.

People are more likely to work hard on their own project than on the boss's project (Prime and Salib 2014b) as a result of two psychological processes. The first one, *implicit egotism*, is the notion that we tend to like things that we identify with or that remind us of ourselves. When employees feel like they're working on a project that they've envisioned, they identify more with it and they tend to put in more time and energy to make it successful. The second process is referred to as the *endowment effect*. We tend to highly value what we have simply because it's ours—evident in studies in which people are given an item as theirs and then are asked to trade it for a more valuable one. Most people choose not to make the trade because they become attached to the first item. When it comes to work situations, employees feel a great attachment to specific tasks or projects that the boss has given them as theirs, and they're more likely to work hard on them.

Third, humble leaders tend to be more liked by others. As human beings, we move away from others who self-promote and are self-aggrandizing, but we're generally attracted to leaders who tend to listen to us and who are humble about their abilities. As a result, humble leaders tend to have more interpersonal influence and can induce others to work harder to achieve organizational goals (Prime and Salib 2014a). In the next section, we explore the empirical research behind these arguments.

5

Let's start by taking a look at some of the general studies on humility. First, not surprisingly, the evidence shows that humble people are more likely to help others than nonhumble people. In one university study, participants listened to a recorded interview in which another student talked about his need for help. They were then presented with the opportunity to help that student by volunteering their time. Separately, the same participants were asked to examine a list of traits and to associate as quickly as possible humility or arrogance traits with themselves or with others. The idea was that a humble person should more quickly associate *humble* than *arrogant* with herself, and the other way round. Terms related to humility included *humble, modest, tolerant, down-to-earth, respectful,* and *open-minded,* whereas arrogance-related terms included *arrogant, immodest, egotistical, high-and-mighty, closed-minded,* and *conceited.* Participants who fell into the high-humility group volunteered significantly more time to help their fellow students than did participants in the low-humility group (LaBouff et al. 2011).

Other research has also shown that people who behave modestly in response to their own performance tend to be better liked than those who behave boastfully and that arrogant people are generally less admired than modest people. Arrogant presenters, for example, tend to be less effective than others, whereas those who display some modesty tend to receive the best evaluations from their peers (Bond, Leung, and Wan 1982; Hareli and Weiner 2000).

Being dominant and arrogant also has some negative health effects. This evidence has emerged from studies concerning, of all things, male baboons. In the wild, alpha males are the most dominant baboons. They do what they want, and they don't answer to anyone. Beta males, on the other hand, tend to avoid conflict and confrontation. Researchers measured stress hormone levels in both types of animals by analyzing their fecal samples. They discovered that alpha male baboons have much higher levels of cortisol, a stress hormone, than beta male ones. Alpha males have significantly more cortisol because they constantly need to protect their status as lead baboons by fighting other males and by following their mates to fend off approaches by other males. Beta males, on the other hand, were less stressed because they were not concerned with fending off other males, although they ended up mating with the same number of females as their alpha counterparts (Gesquire et al. 2011). Similarly, among humans, there is increasing evidence that people who are more humble tend to enjoy better physical and mental health than those who are less humble. Data from a recent nationwide survey show that humility can act as a buffer between significant life events and happiness and life satisfaction. This result implies that humble people are better able to navigate life's major stressors without serious effects on their quality of life (Krausea et al. 2016).

Moreover, a growing body of research shows significant advantages to being humble in individual and group settings. In one study set up in an undergraduate management class, students completed individual assignments and tests and worked in groups on a 10-week project. Each group member was asked to confidentially rate his teammates on a humility test. The findings showed that students who had higher humility ratings tended to do better on individual course requirements and contributed more to their team's performance.

But the most intriguing finding was that humility mattered more for people who had relatively lower mental abilities. Being humble made a considerable difference for people with lower intelligence levels but had only a small positive effect on performance among smart people. The authors explain that "measures of raw general mental ability may reflect cognitive processing speed and the ability to grasp new concepts. But the ability to learn isn't the same thing as a willingness to learn. General mental ability says little about how willing someone is to seek and apply critical feedback, admit mistakes, and benefit from the positive modeling of others. Humble people with lower general mental ability may still perform well because they may be more willing to enact these learning behaviors to master performance tasks" (Owens, Johnson, and Mitchell 2013, 1527). When assessing an individual's performance improvement over time (difference in test scores between the first exam and the final exam, for example), humility was the strongest predictor of improvement—much stronger than self-efficacy, conscientiousness, and general mental ability. These findings clearly indicate that humility isn't just about appearances. Humble people perform better because they are more receptive to feedback, make better informed decisions based on accurate self-views, and are more appreciative of and receptive to others' strengths.

A later study set in a similar environment showed positive associations between collective humility and team growth and performance. Here, the students worked in teams on a multistage computer simulation in the context of car manufacturing. The simulation required the teams to make multiple strategic decisions and to compete for market share and stock value. Halfway through the exercise, the students independently rated their team on collective humility and team growth climate. The results showed that more humble teams were more likely to attain their ambitions and achieve the success that they hoped for and were also more likely to triple their stock price by the end of the simulation (Owens and Hekman 2016).

Moving away from experimental inquiries, organizational research is starting to examine humility among employees. For example, in a sample of assisted living staff who provided support to challenging customers needing medical care, the participants were asked to rate themselves on six personality traits. Their supervisors also rated them on important job skills. The results showed that those that rated themselves high on humility (along with honesty) received higher scores on performance by their supervisors. The fact that humility predicted job performance much more than any other personality trait—such as emotionality, extraversion, agreeableness, conscientiousness, and openness to experience—is also worth noting (Johnson, Rowatt, and Petrini 2011).

6

Let's turn our attention now to leaders. The introduction of humility into leadership studies can be credited to Jim Collins (2001) and his best-selling management book *Good to Great*. Collins and his team identified 11 companies that made the transition from good financial performance to great financial performance. These companies first had cumulative stock returns at or below the general stock market. After a certain transition point, the companies had cumulative returns of at least three times the market average over a period of 15 years. The researchers set out to identify the common characteristics among these companies and what differentiated them from comparison companies in the same industry that failed to make similar transitions. Of the many principles Collins identifies, *Level 5 leadership* is the one that stands out the most (Collins 2001).

To better understand Level 5 leadership, it's important to explain what the other levels mean.

- Level 1 leader: Makes productive contributions through talent, knowledge, skills, and good work habits
- Level 2 leader: Contributes to her team by working effectively with others
- Level 3 leader: Competently manages and organizes people and resources to achieve effective and efficient outcomes
- Level 4: Effectively creates a compelling vision and motivates the group to reach high levels of performance
- Level 5: Possesses Level 1 through Level 4 traits, but also demonstrates humility and determination

All 11 companies that transformed from good to great performance were headed by Level 5 leaders. Collins (2001, 12) and his team "were surprised, really shocked, to discover the type of leadership required for turning a good company into a great one." He notes, "Compared to high-profile leaders with big personalities, who make headlines and become celebrities, the good-to-great leaders seem to have come from Mars. Self-effacing, quiet, reserved and even shy—these leaders are a paradoxical blend of personal humility and professional will" (Collins 2001, 12–13).

This puzzling combination of humility and resolve was best displayed by a little-known CEO named Darwin Smith. Smith grew up as a poor farm boy, putting himself through college and finally earning a law degree from Harvard University. He then joined

Kimberly-Clark, a longstanding paper company, as the in-house lawyer. Smith was hardworking and very shy. In a move that surprised many, the board appointed him to be CEO in 1971. Even Smith himself wasn't sure it was the right decision. In retrospect, it turned out to be a brilliant one—Smith remained the CEO of Kimberly-Clark for 20 years, during which he turned it into the leading paper-based consumer products company in the world.

When Collins and his team studied Smith's leadership style at Kimberly-Clark, what struck them was his fierce resolve. He always did what he thought was right. Shortly after being appointed as CEO, he concluded, along with his team, that the coated paper business—the company's traditional core product—couldn't survive the economy and the competition. Smith decided to sell the paper mills and focus resources instead into consumer products, such as Kleenex and Huggies. He even closed the mill in Kimberly, Wisconsin, a town named after the company. The business media and Wall Street analysts vehemently questioned the move. But Smith never faltered—he believed that it was the right strategy for his organization. In the following years, Kimberly-Clark's cumulative stock returns reached 4.1 times the market return, easily outperforming its main competitors, Scott Paper and Procter & Gamble.

Throughout his years as CEO, Smith never believed his own hype. At his retirement, he reflected on his career and modestly stated, "I never stopped trying to become qualified for the job" (Collins 2001, 20). The other executives in the good-to-great companies displayed similar behaviors in interviews by Collins's team. When asked by the researchers about their contributions, they would say something like, "I hope I am not sounding like a big shot" or "Did I have a lot to do with it? Oh, that sounds so self-serving, I don't think I can take much credit. We were blessed with marvelous people" (Collins 2001, 27). But this approach wasn't the type of false modesty or "humblebragging" that we often see today (more on that later on in chapter 8). It wasn't just pretending to be humble—this was humility in action that was noticed by everyone around. When these leaders' colleagues were asked to describe them, they used terms such as *humble, modest, gracious, self-effacing,* and *understated.*

The key idea here is that these leaders achieved greatness for their companies, not despite of, but *because* of their humility. They did it by combining humility with an unwavering professional will. While they demonstrated a compelling modesty and shunned public adulation, they also produced superb results. They acted with quiet, calm determination and relied heavily on standards, not sheer charisma, to inspire others. They did what was needed to produce long-term results, despite difficulties and skepticism. When apportioning credit for the company's success, they looked beyond themselves, to others, external factors, and good luck. But when assigning responsibility for bad performance, they looked in the mirror and took the full blame. Toward the end of their reigns, they worked diligently to set up their successors for future success, and they channeled their ambition to forge enduringly great companies (Collins 2001).

These findings provided empirical evidence of what many have suspected for a long time: Humility, ambition, and high performance are related to each other. Despite the subsequent failures of some of the companies included in Collins's sample (e.g., Fannie Mae, Circuit City, Wells Fargo), Collins's point is that humble leaders with great determination can lead their organization to high performance, a point confirmed by subsequent research (Hamilton and Knoche 2007).

What is glaringly missing from Collins's and others' analyses is an explanation of how humility and performance are actually connected. Recent research is starting to clarify that connection. One way leader humility can affect outcomes is through employee engagement and satisfaction. In a study of a large midwestern health services organization, several hundred employees were asked to rate the humility of their immediate supervisors. They were also asked to assess their own job engagement and satisfaction. Participants who viewed their leaders as humble were more likely to report being happy at work and less likely to voluntarily leave the organization.

"In contrast to 'rousing' employees through charismatic, energetic, and idealistic leadership approaches . . . , our study suggests a 'quieter' leadership approach, with listening, being transparent about limitations, and appreciating follower strengths and contributions as effective ways to engage employees," remark the authors (Owens, Johnson, and Mitchell 2013, 1531).

In the current competitive labor market, organizations compete to attract and retain talent, and many high performers leave their jobs when they don't feel as if their bosses listen to them or recognize their potential. Humility, then, could be a valuable tool for attracting and retaining talented employees. Moreover, other evidence shows that leader humility can help followers better express their personality and individual innovation in the workplace. A recent report that surveyed more than 1,500 workers from Australia, China, Germany, India, Mexico, and the United States found that when employees observed acts of humility among their managers, they were more likely to report feeling included in their work teams (Prime and Salib 2014a).

Leader humility also helps to create a culture of shared unpretentiousness that enables the team to grow and reach its full potential. In another study of health services teams, employees examined their leader's humility in terms of whether he's willing to learn from others, admits not knowing something, and compliments others on their strengths. Teams that perceived their leaders to be better on these behaviors had higher collective humility, team growth, and performance (Owens and Hekman 2016). These findings provide empirical evidence for the old advice to lead by example. It turns out that when leaders behave humbly, employees emulate their humble behaviors, thus creating collective humility. This atmosphere enables the team to achieve its potential, which ultimately enhances performance.

The notion that humble leaders can help create an organization-wide culture of humility has also been endorsed by research. The humility of the CEO, of other executives, and of employees can result in an emphasis on cultures, systems, procedures, and structures aimed at developing organizational humility. This type of shared humility allows an openness to new paradigms, eagerness to learn from others, acknowledgment of limitations and mistakes, and more realistic understanding of the organization and its environment. Management researchers Dusya Vera and Antonio Rodriguez-Lopez argue that organizational humility is the "cornerstone of organizational learning, high-quality service to customers and employees, and organizational resilience" (Vera and Rodriguez-Lopez 2004, 393). Therefore, humility doesn't just lead to everyone feeling good about themselves—it can be a significant advantage for the organization in relation to its competitors.

The last study linking leader humility to performance that we'll examine comes to us from Chinese private companies. More than 60 CEOs were interviewed, and data were gathered from more than one thousand top management team members and middle managers. The qualities of a humble CEO, as defined by the study, included self-awareness, openness to feedback, appreciation of others, low self-focus, and appreciation of the greater good. Humble leaders were more able to empower their top and middle managers to collaborate, share information, make joint decisions, and develop a shared vision. Through their humility, CEOs won acceptance from their followers by appealing to collective interests and downplaying strong ego dominance. This evidence challenges the view held by some that humble CEOs lack confidence or aren't able to motivate their employees. Because humble CEOs willingly admit both strengths and weaknesses and are appreciative of others' strengths, they demonstrate vast self-confidence that can help them win others over. As suggested by the study's authors, we need to start thinking differently about leader influence: "There is a misconception that influential leaders should be masculine, dominant, and authoritarian. Those views suggest that leadership requires a strong personal desire for influence. But this overlooks the second piece of the influence puzzle: leadership also depends on whether subordinates accept leaders' influence. Research shows that bold and assertive leaders who lack genuine concern for others undermine their influence on subordinates" (Ou et al. 2014, 60).

The research discussed in this section strongly suggests that humbitious leaders achieve more success for themselves, their teams, and their organizations than arrogant ones do. Leader humility, when combined with strength and ambition, has a clear positive effect across all levels and helps empower and uplift employees. In the next section, we'll see how one healthcare leader has used humility to bring people together and enhance organizational performance.

7

The new system CEO was yelling and screaming, slamming his fists on the conference room table. His eyes were bulging, nostrils flaring. And then the f-bombs starting raining down, one after the other, directed at everyone and everything. The three hospital CEOs were stunned. They had been in their positions for a few years now, a tight group of small hospital leaders. Their previous system CEO was nothing like this. But ever since their organization was acquired by a new company, things had taken a turn for the worse.

After the meeting, Ed Lamb, one of the small hospital leaders, was dismayed by the tone of the new system CEO. He decided that something needed to be done, so he set up a private meeting. In the meeting, he told his new boss, in a diplomatic way, that his language was offensive and that the culture of the organization wasn't compatible with his aggressive approach. The system CEO just stared back at him in silence. A week later, at the next executive meeting, the system CEO picked up from where he left off—but this time he was directing his venom straight at Ed. After the umpteenth insult, Ed couldn't take it anymore. He walked out of the room. Right after the meeting, the system CEO called Ed to his office. He berated Ed and accused him of being insubordinate, of not being a team player. In a couple of weeks, when the insults started coming at yet another executive meeting, Ed thought to himself, "I can't take this anymore. I am not a good fit here." He resigned and went to work for another hospital system (Lamb 2016).

Today, Ed is the former Chairman of the American College of Healthcare Executives and the CEO of Mount Carmel Health System in Columbus, Ohio. He recalls a few other times in his career when he had to deal with loud, disrespectful bosses. These experiences have helped mold him into the humble, respectful leader that he is now. "The yeller and screamer kind are insecure; they use intimidation and fear tactics," he observes. "They might get things done in the short term, but people won't stay long term; they are not motivated to bring others to help achieve the vision. But when you create an environment where you are approachable, you can get things done. People are comfortable coming to you to talk about everything, about problems, which has a huge effect on outcomes. They won't be worried, walking on eggshells. They can come and tell you, 'I don't know how to do this,' and you can say, 'Let's get others involved and get things done'" (Lamb 2016).

According to Ed, to be an effective leader, you have to have a clear vision and understanding of what you want to accomplish. But you also have to admit that you don't know everything. Just as we saw earlier with the five foundations, humility is about being willing to admit this fact to others and to ask for their input. Ed explains to his team what the end goal is and that there are many ways to get there. Then he tasks them with finding the best moral and ethical approach. If he makes a suggestion and other team members think it won't work, he doesn't get upset, shout, and yell. Instead, he asks them to help him understand why his idea is wrong and he tries to find a better way to move forward.

Ed's views are supported by my survey of healthcare organizations. I surveyed 577 employees, supervisors, directors, and executives working in nine different hospital and health systems. When asked which traits of leaders have negatively influenced their own careers, arrogant came in the first place, with a response rate of 52 percent. For many respondents, nothing has been more damaging to their careers than having an arrogant boss. Similarly, when considering traits of leaders who have been the least successful at improving organizational outcomes and getting things done, self-focused came in second place (44 percent) and arrogant came in fourth place (42 percent). According to these results, not only do self-focused and arrogant leaders frustrate and disengage their followers, but they may also drive their organizations into poor performance. (See the appendix at the end of the book for the complete results of the survey.)

In Greek mythology, Narcissus was known for extraordinary beauty and astounding physique. He was loved by gods and humans alike, but he rarely reciprocated that love. A young man named Aminias was one of his unrequited lovers. According to the myth, poor Aminias killed himself on Narcissus's doorstep while praying to the gods to punish Narcissus for all the pain that he had caused. Shortly after, Narcissus found himself by a river. He stopped for a drink and saw his own reflection in the water. He was surprised by his own beauty and instantly fell in love with his image. Unable to obtain the object of his desire, he was punished by the gods and suffered a miserable death at the banks of the river (Guerber 2012).

The myth of Narcissus is one of the most popular stories about the dangers of being self-absorbed. Sigmund Freud (1914), the father of psychoanalysis, was inspired by the story to identify a personality disorder associated with self-infatuation called *narcissism*. In his remarkable essay "On Narcissism," he defines the disorder as a form of neurosis in which the person adores himself. Freud postulates that narcissism develops when an individual turns the affection that is typically directed toward other objects back on himself. This reversal typically happens because the individual is unable to express love to others and have it expressed back to him. As a result, he suffers from low self-esteem, shame, guilt, and lack of interest in others. Building on this conception, narcissism has been defined by psychologists as a personality trait characterized by a sense of personal superiority and grandiosity and a desire for power, attention, and confirmation. Because of their lack of empathy, narcissists engage in exploitative behaviors, often taking credit for someone else's work and blaming mistakes on others. When confronted with negative feedback or criticism, they turn aggressive and hostile (Bogart, Benotsch, and Pavlovic 2004).

Narcissism is measured by the Narcissistic Personality Inventory (NPI), a validated instrument. The test consists of 40 pairs of statements, and for each pair the respondent selects the one that best reflects her personality. Examples of statement pairs include "When people compliment me I sometimes get embarrassed" versus "I know that I am good because everybody keeps telling me so." Another example that is related to leadership is "I'm a born leader" versus "Leadership is a quality that takes a long time to develop" (Raskin and Terry 1988). I recently took the NPI online and was happy to receive a score of 14 out 40, which is lower than the average for US adults, 15.3 (yes, I'm aware of the irony of bragging about being humble!). The NPI is broken down into five main categories: authority, self-sufficiency, superiority, exhibitionism, exploitativeness, vanity, and entitlement. I scored the lowest on vanity and entitlement, while my highest score was on superiority—not something I'm particularly proud of. The NPI is sometimes used in organizations to measure CEO narcissism. But in situations in which that isn't possible, leader narcissism can be measured, for example, by assessing the prominence of the CEO's picture in annual reports, the use of the first person ("I") by the CEO in interviews, the status of the CEO in press releases, and the compensation of the CEO compared to that of other executives (Pfeffer 2015).

The overlap between narcissistic behaviors and some leaders' behaviors is obvious. As we discussed in the previous chapter, most well-regarded CEOs have narcissistic traits: Steve Jobs of Apple, Jack Welch of General Electric, Michael Eisner of Disney, and Elon Musk of Tesla and SpaceX. Consider the example of Larry Ellison, the founder and former CEO of Oracle, a computer technology company. Ellison is one of the richest people on the planet, and he does everything that you would expect a celebrity CEO to do. He owns mansions around the world and has a large collection of luxury cars. He commissioned a massive yacht. He jumps headfirst into extreme sports such as mountain biking and body surfing, and he's a licensed pilot who owns two military jets. He has been married and divorced four times, and it's said that he has dated as many as three of his employees at the same time (Kim 2015).

In 2003, Oracle was involved in a hostile takeover bid for People-Soft, another software company. The companies were fighting each other in courts and through advertisements when their respective CEOs started exchanging jabs in the press. PeopleSoft's CEO, Craig Conway, described the takeover situation as, "It's like me asking if I could buy your dog so I can go out back and shoot it." To this, Ellison replied, "[He] thought I was going to shoot his dog. I love animals. If Craigy [Conway] and his dog were standing next to each other and, trust me, I had one bullet, it wouldn't be for the dog" (Finkelstein, Whitehead, and Campbell 2009, 144).

Ellison is the poster child for the narcissist leader. In one of the most famous quotes in the history of corporate America, an Oracle employee is supposed to have declared, "The difference between God and Larry is that God does not believe he is Larry." A book by that title appeared shortly thereafter (Wilson 2003). All extravagances aside, however, Ellison was a very successful CEO. He founded Oracle with $1,200 of his own money and turned it into a billion-dollar multinational giant. This blend of personal characteristics might make us wonder about the personal and organizational success of narcissist leaders—do narcissist leaders succeed because of, or despite, their narcissistic traits?

In his remarkable *Harvard Business Review* essay on narcissism, psychoanalyst and leadership expert Michael Maccoby labels leaders such as Ellison *productive narcissists*. He notes that these are gifted strategists who can see the big picture and aren't afraid to push the envelope. "Indeed, one reason we look to productive narcissists in times of great transition is that they have the audacity to push through the massive transformations that society periodically undertakes. Productive narcissists are not only risk takers willing to get the job done, but also charmers who can convert the masses with their rhetoric," he observed (Maccoby 2004). However, because these leaders lack self-knowledge and don't have any restraint(s), they may turn into unproductive dreamers. When their plans don't pan out, they blame the circumstances, or their enemies, instead of looking at themselves and learning from their own mistakes. "This tendency toward grandiosity and distrust is the Achilles' heel of narcissism," notes Maccoby (2004). In another brilliant essay titled "The Dark Side of Charisma," psychologists Robert Hogan, Robert Raskin, and Dan Fazzini note that narcissists are terrible managers because they "are biased to take more credit for success than is legitimate, and biased to avoid acknowledging responsibility for their failures and shortcomings for the same reasons that they claim more success than is their due" (Hogan, Raskin, and Fazzini 1990, 636). This behavior is diametrically opposed to that of Level 5 leaders.

Examined through the lens of leadership, narcissists have many serious flaws. Even the most productive narcissists are extremely sensitive to criticisms, "almost unimaginably thin-skinned" (Maccoby 2004). They aren't interested in hearing what others think of them, and they can be abrasive with dissenting followers. While they claim that they value teamwork, what they really mean is they want a team of yes-men who never question their decisions. Moreover, narcissistic leaders are generally poor listeners. Maccoby tells the story of one narcissistic CEO who hired him to assess his leadership approach. He allowed Maccoby to interview his immediate team and report back to him on what they were thinking. After collecting the data, Maccoby reported the results to the CEO. He described the exchange that took place: "'So what do they think of me?' he asked with seeming nonchalance as we walked together. 'They think you are very creative and courageous,' I told him, 'but they also feel that you don't listen.' 'Excuse me, what did you say?' he shot back at once, pretending not to hear. His response was humorous, but it was also tragic. In a very real way, this CEO could not hear my criticism because it was too painful to tolerate" (Maccoby 2004).

Most narcissistic leaders believe that they didn't reach success by listening to others and including them in decisions. While they crave understanding, they tend to score very low on empathy themselves. They don't care where others are coming from and aren't interested in listening to other people's emotions. For example, one narcissistic CEO in Maccoby's study noted, "If I listened to my employees' needs and demands, they would eat me alive" (Maccoby 2004). Narcissistic leaders can be brutally exploitative and are often not liked by their followers. Not surprisingly, they don't like to be mentored and don't have any patience for mentoring others. Even when they occasionally take on mentees, they tend to instruct rather than coach them, hoping that the learners will become pale reflections of themselves. Also, because they're ultracompetitive, narcissistic leaders will stop at nothing to win, which creates a dangerous environment of warfare and mistrust. Driven by their fears and suspicions, they mistakenly find enemies among their most loyal followers and, in the process, end up driving their organizations into the ground.

8

Organizational research lends some support to the previously mentioned views, although the evidence is generally mixed. When studying the relationship between narcissism and leadership, researchers typically distinguish between two phenomena: leadership emergence (whether someone gets a leadership position or is selected for it) and leadership effectiveness (once in a leadership position, the degree to which the individual is effective in the role) (Grijalva et al. 2015). Let's look first at whether narcissists tend to be chosen for leadership positions. In order to be selected for such a position, one has to be noticed and remembered. Managers tend to select people who promote themselves and draw attention to their own positive qualities and past accomplishments. Job candidates who engage in more self-promotion tend to receive better evaluations from interviewers and tend to be selected more often for hiring. Narcissists are typically very confident, which presents a huge advantage for their emergence as leaders. Research in experimental settings shows that overconfident individuals achieve higher status, respect, and influence in groups, even after teammates have been shown evidence of those overconfident individuals' poor performance. In fact, many of the narcissist's natural characteristics, such as social dominance and extraversion, are viewed by others as leader-like traits (Anderson et al. 2012).

When individuals who don't know each other are assigned to work in groups with no formal leader designation, narcissists invariably emerge as leaders regardless of their individual performance. For example, in a study of managers participating in a leaderless group discussion exercise, narcissists were singled out as leaders by their teammates, as well as by a group of independent experts who had received extensive training in rating leadership.

However—and this finding is critical—once team members interact over a longer period and become more familiar with the actions of the narcissistic leaders, they don't perceive them as effective leaders anymore (Brunell et al. 2008; Nevicka, Baas, and Ten Velden 2016). This effect is often referred to in the management literature as the *chocolate cake model.* "Relationships with narcissistic leaders can be a paradoxical experience, much like eating chocolate cake," write Chin Wei Ong and colleagues in a recent article. "The first bite of chocolate cake is usually rich in flavor and texture, and extremely gratifying. After a while, however, the richness of this flavor makes one feel increasingly nauseous. Being led by a narcissist could be a similar experience: Narcissists might initially be perceived as effective leaders, but these positive perceptions may decrease over time" (Ong et al. 2015, 237). In another experiment, narcissistic individuals were initially described by others as "confident, entertaining, and physically attractive," but toward the end they were referred to as "hostile, arrogant, and cold" (Paulhus 1998, 1204).

The question of whether narcissism is good or bad for leadership effectiveness is one of the longest-running issues in the research literature (Campbell et al. 2011). Timothy Judge, Jeffrey LePine, and Bruce Louis Rich (2006) found that, in one study, narcissism had a positive effect on leadership effectiveness, as rated by others, but in another study, it had a negative effect. Narcissists are more likely to adopt bold visions that create significant organizational change, according to some, but they are negligent in pursuing stakeholder-oriented visions that inspire followers, according to others. High scores on psychopathic traits such as feeling grandiose and lacking remorse and empathy are associated with perceptions of good communication skills, strategic thinking, and creative or innovative ability and, at the same time, are strongly related to poor management styles, the failure to act as a team player, and poor performance appraisals (Brown and Treviño 2006; De Luque et al. 2008). Narcissistic CEOs in a study of high-technology manufacturing companies were found to be more entrepreneurial and aggressive in their strategic actions, which resulted in more variability in each firm's performance over time (i.e., performance increases as well as decreases). In these unstable situations, media and popular culture analysts tend to focus more on positive rather than negative performance and are likely to give these CEOs disproportionate credit for performance gains (Wales, Patel, and Lumpkin 2013).

One of the few examples of strong support for the effectiveness of narcissistic leaders comes from a study of 392 CEOs of large companies during the economic crisis of 2007. At the onset of the crisis, firms with highly narcissistic CEOs witnessed a greater decline in performance, possibly because these leaders are less likely to protect against potential shocks. However, these same companies significantly increased their performance after the crisis as a result of their CEOs' abilities to make hard decisions that allowed them to recover from setbacks. Ironically, this outcome may have to do with narcissistic CEOs' lack of empathy (Patel and Cooper 2014). "In times of radical change," Maccoby notes, "lack of empathy can actually be a strength. A narcissist finds it easier than other personality types to buy and sell companies, to close and move facilities, and to lay off employees—decisions that inevitably make many people angry and sad" (Maccoby 2004). Narcissistic leaders may also view these crises as a threat to their own egos, which can help fuel their future performance.

If you find all this research confusing, don't feel bad—the evidence varies greatly. More recent research, however, seems to provide more clarity. A comprehensive study of more than 1,900 individuals with leadership responsibilities in six companies measured effectiveness in terms of supervisor reports, subordinate reports, and peer reports (typically referred to as a 360-degree evaluation). The results showed that the narcissism–leadership effectiveness relationship looks like an inverted U shape, which means that very low and very high levels of narcissism actually lead to poor performance. Only moderate levels of narcissism are positively related to effectiveness (Grijalva et al. 2015). Another study of followers and leaders working for a large health insurance organization found somewhat similar results. When narcissistic leaders displayed some evidence of humility, they were rated higher on leadership effectiveness, and their followers were more engaged and performed better on their job tasks (Owens, Wallace, and Waldman 2015).

How can narcissistic leaders be humble, you may ask? Isn't that an oxymoron? Seemingly contradictory personal attributes sometimes exist simultaneously and can work together to produce positive results. For example, while Steve Jobs was known to be a raging narcissist, he showed evidence of humility after returning from exile in his second stint as Apple CEO. The people who worked with him at that time noted that he was more open to suggestions from others, more willing to acknowledge past mistakes, and more appreciative of his executive team members. When the negative aspects of narcissism are tempered by the dimensions of humility, narcissistic leaders are more effective. Bradley Owens, Angela Wallace, and David Waldman (2015, 1205) explain this curious interaction, saying, "Narcissistic tendencies toward exploiting others, being self-absorbed, and demanding admiration are offset by overtly drawing attention to and promoting others' strengths and contributions. A sense of superiority is neutralized by the leader's admissions of limits and mistakes, and self-centered perspectives are transcended or expanded by the leader's being receptive to others' ideas and feedback." Effective leaders, therefore, are those who are paradox savvy: They have a strong sense of self while also maintaining humility. For example, if the leader and her team accomplish a significant task or achieve an important goal, she accepts praise and recognition from her board and colleagues, while at the same time sharing it with the team that made the accomplishment possible (Waldman and Bowen 2016).

Despite the evidence showing the negative effects of narcissism in most situations, many organizations select highly narcissistic individuals for their leadership positions and tend to value them more than humble ones. A recent study by Stanford University professor Charles O'Reilly III and colleagues shows that highly narcissistic CEOs received more than other CEOs in total direct compensation—including salary, bonus, and stock options—and were paid disproportionately relative to other executive team members. However, the firms with CEOs higher in narcissism didn't perform better than those led by CEOs lower in narcissism, which suggests that "shareholder value may be sacrificed for the CEO's narcissistic personality" (O'Reilly et al. 2014, 228). You can't help but notice the hypocrisy in how some organizations appoint their leaders. In public, they say that they want humble executives who put others ahead of themselves, but in reality, they appoint egocentric leaders and pay them generously.

9

Let's look now at a related but different leadership trait: extraversion. Extraversion is a personality trait of those who enjoy the opportunity to be with others, such as participation at social gatherings, and are generally vocal and full of energy. In one of the studies relating to leadership emergence that we discussed earlier, narcissists were more likely to be chosen as leaders by their team members because they were generally extraverted: outgoing, energetic, and dominant (Grijalva et al. 2015). However, if you recall, Level 5 leaders in *Good to Great* were the opposite: introverted, quiet, and even shy. Darwin Smith, for example, was mild mannered and had little interest in joining industry groups or high-profile executive associations. He preferred to spend his vacation alone at his farm (Barboza 1995).

How can we make sense of these seeming contradictions? In this section, I'll explore the question of extraversion and introversion in greater depth.

The notion that human beings have different personality types or preferences comes from the work of Swiss psychiatrist Carl G. Jung. In 1921, Jung postulated that what appears to be random behavior is actually the result of differences in the way people prefer to use their mental capacities. When it comes to mental functions, for example, some people prefer to take in information (*perceive*), whereas other people tend to organize the information and make conclusions (*judge*). Jung also observes that some people are more energized by the external world (*extraversion*), while others are more energized by the internal world (*introversion*) (Jung 1921). Building on Jung's ideas, Isabel Briggs Myers and her mother Katharine Cook Briggs developed an easy-to-use personality test now referred to as the Myers-Briggs Type Indicator (MBTI) personality inventory. In addition to perceiving (P) versus judging (J) and extraversion (E) versus introversion (I), Myers and Briggs consider two additional personality dimensions. In relation to information processing, they call the preference to focus on the basic information *sensing* (S) and referred to the preference to interpret and add meaning as *intuition* (N). When making decisions, the inclination to consider logic and consistency is labelled *thinking* (T), whereas a penchant for considering people and special circumstances is called *feeling* (F) (Myers-Briggs Foundation 2017).

Most people know their MBTI type and spend time reflecting on it and discussing it with others. Of all the personality preferences, introversion versus extraversion probably gets the most attention from experts and the general public, although many people don't clearly understand what these labels mean. Recent research on personalities has helped clarify some of the confusion. People often believe that extraverts get their energy from social interactions, whereas introverts get it from reflecting on their thoughts and feelings. The evidence indicates, however, that this isn't the case. Introverts and extraverts spend about the same amount of time interacting with others and experience the same increase in energy when talking with them. When people rate their energy in a given period, both introverts and extraverts attribute the energizing hours to those that involve interaction with others. So what makes introverts and extraverts different from each other? Mainly sensitivity to stimulation. Introverts are more prone to being overstimulated by intense or prolonged social interaction and by loud events or dangerous activities such as parties or skydiving. While extraverts enjoy that overstimulation, introverts prefer to retreat to a quiet place to recharge (Fleeson, Malanos, and Achille 2002; Pavot, Diener, and Fujita 1990).

Another common misconception is that all introverts are bad public speakers. While introverts do suffer slightly more anxiety before speeches and presentations, research shows that most of the anxiety related to speaking is unrelated to introversion and extraversion. More relevant factors include whether the person is more anxious in general, whether she thinks the audience is nice or hostile, and whether she believes that she'll do a good or bad job on that particular topic. The evidence is that everyone, including introverts, can learn, through practice and rehearsing, to control their anxiety and to become better performers (MacIntyre and Thivierge 1995; Stelmack 2004). Malcolm Gladwell, a well-known author and introvert who has to give plenty of talks while promoting his books, notes that "speaking is not an act of extraversion, it has nothing to do with extraversion. It's a performance, and many performers are hugely introverted" (Gladwell 2010).

People often think that because of their outgoing personalities, extraverts are much better than introverts at connecting with others and building networks. But, here again, the evidence is stacked up against extraverts. Several studies involving individuals working in groups indicate that extraverts produce more negative emotions in others, have more trouble in relationships with their teammates, and initially may be accorded a higher status but tend to lose that over time (similar to the chocolate cake phenomenon we discussed in section 9) (Eisenkraft and Elfenbei 2010; Klein et al. 2004). When rated by others, extraverts are typically perceived as overbearing and as engaging in rowdy behaviors that annoy others (Bendersky and Shah 2013). When people feel negatively about you and are bothered by your actions, it's hard to build and maintain long-term relationships and sustain meaningful networks.

10

This interest in personality types can be traced back to the rise of industrial America, when people left small towns, where everyone knew everyone else, and arrived in large cities, where they needed to make impressions on complete strangers. The idea of having a good personality, in fact, didn't become common until the twentieth century. The cultural historian Warren Susman refers to this as the shift from the *culture of character* to the *culture of personality*. In the culture of character, when most people lived among others who knew them and knew their parents, the ideal person was serious, disciplined, and honorable. What counted was not the impression you made in public, but how you acted in private with those who knew you. In today's culture of personality, we constantly meet new people and worry about how others perceive us. In this reality where everyone constantly needs to perform, we're captivated by people who are bold and entertaining (Susman 1984).

This rise of the extravert ideal—"the omnipresent belief that the ideal self is gregarious, alpha, and comfortable in the spotlight"— affects many of our practices and organizations in the contemporary era (Cain 2015). Most people would argue that, all things equal, being extraverted is considerably better than being introverted. Consider, for example, the educational field. The majority of teachers at all school levels prefer extraverted students and reward them with better grades and more attention, whereas the introverted are often overlooked or considered shy or antisocial (Godsey 2015; May 2014). A student who is a good listener and who gives one good reflective comment is considered too quiet, whereas one who constantly raises his hand is celebrated. In a widely publicized blog post a few years ago, high school English teacher Natalie Munro mused about what she wished she could write on her students' report cards. She had especially harsh words for introverted kids: "She just sits there emotionless for an entire 90 minutes, staring into the abyss, never volunteering to speak or do anything" and "Shy isn't cute in 11th grade; it's annoying. Must learn to advocate for himself instead of having Mommy do it" (Canning and Katrandjian 2011). The comments received serious backlash and led to the teacher's eventual suspension, but they reflected deeply rooted attitudes about quiet kids. Classroom environments are more and more often designed to encourage extraverted behavior through desk pods, social learning activities, and group assignments. While these approaches have a lot of merit, the evidence shows that exclusive focus on them can weaken the learning of students who tend to perform better when they're working independently and who prefer classrooms that are quieter and more low key. Parents are also guilty of this emphasis on extraversion by pushing their kids to talk more and "be more social." In extreme cases, some parents are sending their introverted children to psychiatrists to "treat" them for their condition (Cain 2017).

Nowhere is this celebration of the outgoing, talkative type more apparent than in business schools and healthcare administration programs. While preparing for her sensational book *Quiet: The Power of Introverts in a World That Can't Stop Talking*, self-confessed introverted author Susan Cain (2013) decided to spend some time at the Harvard Business School (HBS), the mecca of all extraverts, where socializing is an extreme sport. As soon as they start their coursework, Cain observes, HBS students are assigned to teams in which they do the majority of their work throughout the curriculum. Speaking up in small and large groups is always expected, all courses rely heavily on classroom participation, and everyone goes out for group dinners and drinking sessions almost every night. The approach used in my own graduate-level healthcare administration program at Trinity University is very similar (minus the regular drinking). Most courses in the program allocate anywhere between

5 percent and 10 percent of the final grade to classroom participation and contribution, and group projects and team presentations sometimes amount to two-thirds of the grades. From the very first day, students are highly encouraged to participate in class discussions and to work on their public speaking skills. Five years ago, along with my colleagues, I led an effort to conduct periodic performance evaluations that provide feedback to the students on their professional behavior inside and outside the classroom. Here are examples of comments that we gave to some of the quieter students:

> "We encourage you to feel confident to participate more and be more assertive in group settings."

> "Be more confident to share what you know. Stick your neck out!"

> "You don't seem to be as engaged as we would like you to be. Show more energy and participate more in class discussions to show others what skills you have."

While this approach is biased against introverted types, it has been very effective in helping students identify their shortcomings and work on addressing them, so they can be better prepared for the workplace. The reality is that once they start working in healthcare organizations, introverted interns and young administrators are often mistaken for poor performers by their extraverted bosses. Confirmation bias, which refers to the tendency of people to seek out and make sense of evidence that is consistent with their preexisting beliefs, can be at play. When junior executives sit in the corner, observe, and take notes without contributing to the discussion, they don't attract the attention of others. However, when they speak up in meetings, project confidence, and claim competence with enough conviction, others who work with them view them in that light and tend to assume that they know what they're doing and are deserving of a promotion or salary increase.

Business schools and healthcare administration programs, by overemphasizing the importance of being outgoing and speaking up, believe that they're better equipping their graduates for the demands of the workplace. But what if the workplace has it wrong? What if gregarious alpha types don't perform better than quieter ones? These questions are important to consider in light of recent evidence. Experimental and organizational studies are showing that the loudest people don't always have the best ideas. In one exercise in which master of business administration (MBA) students were assigned to work on a new project in a group setting, team members adopted the ideas of the loudest, most extraverted people, even though the introverts often had better insights. Similar to patterns that other research has discovered about narcissists, those who initiate action tend to be seen as leaders, though others in the group may have better and more innovative thoughts. In the workplace, those who win promotions are typically the best presenters, not the ones with the best ideas. Susan Cain observes, "I worry that there are people who are put in positions of authority because they're good talkers, but they don't have good ideas. It's so easy to confuse schmoozing ability with talent. Someone seems like a good presenter, easy to get along with, and those traits are rewarded. Well, why is that? They're valuable traits, but we put too much of a premium on presenting and not enough on substance and critical thinking" (Cain 2013, 52).

One particular piece of research on leadership extraversion is deserving of our attention. Adam Grant, Francesca Gino, and David A. Hofmann (2011) hypothesize that whether extraverted or introverted leaders are more successful depends on the situation and personality types of their followers. In one study, the researchers analyze data from five big pizza chains. When employees were passive types who did their jobs without exercising initiative, extraverted store managers had weekly profits 16 percent higher than those of introverted managers. However, when employees actively tried to improve work procedures by taking the initiative and making suggestions, the stores managed by introverted leaders outperformed those of extraverted leaders by 14 percent. In another study, college students were divided into competing teams charged with folding T-shirts. The challenge was to fold as many T-shirts as possible in ten minutes. Without telling the students, the research team inserted two actors. In some teams, the actors were instructed to behave passively. In other teams, they were instructed to make suggestions, such as calling a friend who may know a better way to fold the T-shirts. The active actors told their leaders, "Let's call my friend, it will only take a minute or two to teach you how to fold the T-shirt in a better way, do you want to try it?" (Grant, Gino, and Hoffman 2011, 539). Teams with introverted leaders who were more likely to listen to the suggestion and follow it had 24 percent better performance than those with extraverted ones. But when the actors behaved passively and didn't make any suggestions, the teams with extraverted leaders performed better by 22 percent (Grant, Gino, and Hofmann 2011).

These studies indicate that introverts are especially good at leading initiative-takers because of their inclination to listen to others and their ability to restrain themselves from dominating social situations. They're more likely to hear and implement suggestions. Followers perceive these leaders to be more open and receptive to their ideas, which in turn motivates them to work harder. Extraverts, on the other hand, can be so insistent on dominating the conversation that they risk losing their followers' good ideas and may cause them to fall into passivity. Because the majority of professionals in healthcare organizations can be characterized as proactive initiative-takers, an introverted leadership style may be more suitable in that setting.

Given this evidence, it's not surprising that many highly successful CEOs and innovators, such as Darwin Smith, are introverts. Warren Buffett, Charles Schwab, Steven Spielberg, and Brenda Barnes, among others, are all described as shy individuals who prefer to spend time by themselves. Barnes, the former CEO of consumer goods company Sara Lee, admitted, "I've always been shy. People wouldn't call me that, but I am" (Williams 2011, 578). She constantly turned down invitations to give media interviews. While well-established CEOs such as Barnes can openly talk about their introversion, many junior executives don't want others to know about this aspect of their personality. Older polls suggest that more than two-thirds of executives viewed introversion as a liability for leaders, and only 6 percent viewed it as an advantage (Jones 2006).

But there are signs that things are starting to change and the stigma around introversion is slowly disappearing. In his class at Wharton Business School, Adam Grant periodically asks MBA students to raise their hands if they consider themselves introverts. In 2011, only a few hands went up. In 2013, more than one-third of the students admitted to being introverts. But when they completed a confidential survey about their personality preferences, the 2011 and 2013 class members had similar introversion or extraversion scores: about 3.3 on a scale of 1–5 (where 1 is extremely introverted and 5 is extremely extraverted). The number of introverts didn't actually change over the two years—rather, more students became comfortable admitting their introversion to their outgoing class members (Grant 2014).

One of the main reasons behind this change, at least among those business students, is the popularity of the book *Quiet*. Many introverts report that the book has changed their lives and made them comfortable coming out as introverts. More and more executives are also starting to understand that introversion comes with significant strengths, not just liabilities—it's not seen as uninspiring but rather is associated with being calm under pressure, steady, and wise. Cain's call to embrace introversion inspires people beyond management, as well. The successful actress Emma Watson, who played Hermione Granger in the *Harry Potter* movies, recently observed in an interview, "Have you seen *Quiet* by Susan Cain? It discusses how extraverts in our society are bigged up [sic] so much, and if you're anything other than an extravert you're made to think there's something wrong with you. That's like the story of my life. Coming to realize that about myself was very empowering, because I had felt like *Oh my god, there must be something wrong with me, because I don't want to go out and do what all my friends want to do*" (Gevinson 2013).

The discussion about extraversion and introversion naturally leads us to the issue of charisma in leadership. The general public is often captivated by charismatic political leaders, but people working in organizations and leadership researchers have different opinions. When I asked employees and administrators in healthcare organizations about the traits of successful leaders, charisma came in tenth place among 20 traits, with only 27 percent choosing it. (See the appendix at the end of the book for the complete results.) Similarly, management studies have failed to find a relationship between charismatic leaders and objective organizational performance (Agle et al. 2006; Shamir, House, and Arthur 1993). Peter Drucker, the father of management, reflects on this issue: "Among the most effective leaders I have encountered and worked with in a half a century, some locked themselves in their offices and some were ultragregarious. Some were quick and impulsive, while others studied the situation and took forever to come to a decision. The one and only personality trait the effective ones I encountered did have in common was something they did not have: they had little or no 'charisma' and little use either for the term or what it signifies" (Cain 2013, 53).

11

The takeaway is that highly narcissistic leaders are initially chosen more for leadership positions, but their charm seems to wane over time. They can be effective in crisis situations and can energize others with bold visions and strategies, but followers' and organizations' performance tend to suffer under them. Middle ground, where humility is combined with ambition, seems to be the most effective leadership style.

Back to Tony Hsieh, the humbitious CEO of Zappos. Hsieh's humility and determination can be traced back to his teenage years. His parents, first-generation Taiwanese immigrants, stressed academic and musical pursuits but also allowed him to experiment with business ideas. His early ventures consisted of a worm farm, a neighborhood newspaper, and several mail-order businesses. Bolstered by success in the latter, Hsieh decided to invest $800 to sell a magic trick product through a magazine called *Boys' Life*. He was feeling so confident that the idea seemed almost too easy: He calculated that if he received three hundred orders, he would make $2,100 in a short amount of time. "I had discovered the beauty of selling products with high average selling prices and high gross margins," he recalled. But his dream of quick fortunes quickly turned into a nightmare when his new business received no more than one order. "I'd thought that I was the invincible king of mail order, when all that happened was that I had gotten lucky. I learned a valuable lesson in humility," he reflected later (Gelles 2015).

Today, humility guides Hsieh's actions at Zappos, especially in hiring decisions. Frequently named by the media as one of the top places to work in the United States, Zappos receives thousands of applications per year. Many experienced, smart, and talented people are turned away if the company determines that they have big egos. Zappos prefers to hire, train, and develop applicants who are modest and sensible. In fact, "Be Humble" is one of the ten much-celebrated core values of the company. It defines how the company thinks of itself and its relationships with other companies: "We believe that no matter what happens, we should always be respectful of everyone. While we celebrate our individual and team successes, we are not arrogant nor do we treat others differently from how we would want to be treated. Instead, we carry ourselves with a quiet confidence, because we believe that in the long run our character will speak for itself" (Zappos 2010). The company urges its employees to be humble when talking about accomplishments and to treat both large and small vendors with the same respect.

REFERENCES

Agle, B., N. Nagarajan, J. Sonnenfeld, and D. Srinivasan. 2006. "Does CEO Charisma Matter? An Empirical Analysis of the Relationships Among Organizational Performance, Environmental

Uncertainty, and Top Management Team Perceptions of CEO Charisma." *Academy of Management Journal* 94 (1): 161–74.

Anderson, C., S. Brion, A. Moore, and J. A. Kennedy. 2012. "A Status-Enhancement Account of Overconfidence." *Journal of Personality and Social Psychology* 103 (4): 718–35.

Aquinas, T. 1917. *Summa Theologiae*, 2nd and rev. ed. New Advent. Published 2016. www.newadvent.org/summa/index.html.

Argandona, A. 2015. "Humility in Management." *Journal of Business Ethics* 132 (1): 63–71.

Barboza, D. 1995. "Darwin E. Smith, 69, Executive Who Remade a Paper Company." *New York Times*. Published December 28. www.nytimes.com/1995/12/28/us/darwin-e-smith-69-executive-who-remade-a-paper-company.html.

Bendersky, C., and N. Shah. 2013. "The Downfall of Extraverts and Rise of Neurotics: The Dynamic Process of Status Allocation in Task Groups." *Academy of Management Journal* 56 (2): 387–406.

Blanchard, K. 2010. *Leading at a Higher Level: Blanchard on How to Be a High Performing Leader*. Upper Saddle River, NJ: Prentice Hall.

Bobb, D. 2013. *Humility: An Unlikely Biography of America's Greatest Virtue*. Nashville, TN: Nelson Books.

Bogart, L. M., E. G. Benotsch, and J. D. Pavlovic. 2004. "Feeling Superior But Threatened: The Relationship of Narcissism to Social Comparison." *Basic and Applied Social Psychology* 26: 35–44.

Bond, M. H., K. Leung, and K. C. Wan. 1982. "The Social Impact of Self-Effacing Attributions: The Chinese Case." *Journal of Social Psychology* 118 (2): 157–66.

Brown, M. E., and L. K. Treviño. 2006. "Ethical Leadership: A Review and Future Directions." *The Leadership Quarterly* 17 (6): 595–616.

Brunell, A., W. Gentry, W. Campbell, B. Hoffman, K. Kuhnert, and K. DeMarree. 2008. "Leader Emergence: The Case of the Narcissistic Leader." *Personal and Social Psychology Bulletin* 34 (12): 1663–76.

Cain, S. 2017. "How Do Teachers Feel About Their Quiet Students?" *Quiet Revolution*. Accessed March 7. www.quietrev .com/how-do-teachers-feel-about-their-quiet-students.

———. 2015. "The Power of Introverts." *Huffington Post*. Published April 18. www.huffingtonpost.com/susan-cain/introverts -_b_1432650.html.

———. 2013. *Quiet: The Power of Introverts in a World That Can't Stop Talking*. New York: Crown Publishing Group.

Campbell, W. K., B. J. Hoffman, S. M. Campbell, and G. Marchisio. 2011. "Narcissism in Organizational Contexts." *Human Resource Management Review* 21 (4): 268–84.

Canning, A., and A. Katrandjian. 2011. "Teacher Defends Insulting Blog Posts About Her Students: 'I Hear the Trash Company Is Hiring.'" ABC News. Published February 16. http://abcnews.go.com/US/pennsylvania-teacher-wrote -insulting-blog-posts-students-suspended/story?id=12929001.

Collins, J. 2001. *Good to Great: Why Some Companies Make the Leap . . . and Others Don't*. New York: HarperCollins Publishers.

De Luque, M., N. T. Washburn, D. A. Waldman, and R. J. House. 2008. "Unrequited Profit: How Stakeholder and Economic Values Relate to Subordinates' Perceptions of Leadership and Firm Performance." *Administrative Science Quarterly* 53 (4): 626–54.

Eisenkraft, N., and H. A. Elfenbei. 2010. "The Way You Make Me Feel: Evidence for Individual Differences in Affective Presence." *Psychological Science* 21 (4): 505–10.

Finkelstein, S., J. Whitehead, and A. Campbell. 2009. *Think Again: Why Good Leaders Make Bad Decisions and How to Keep It from Happening to You*. Boston: Harvard Business Review Press.

Fleeson, W., A. Malanos, and N. Achille. 2002. "An Intra-individual Process Approach to the Relationship Between Extraversion and Positive Affect: Is Acting Extraverted as 'Good' as Being Extraverted?" *Journal of Personality and Social Psychology* 83 (6): 1409–22.

Freud, S. 1914. "On Narcissism: An Introduction." Semantic Scholar. No date. https://pdfs.semanticscholar.org/4573/39 422536b54a4262a2e26bf0ca6fc4c3b7a9.pdf.

Gelles, D. 2015. "At Zappos, Pushing Shoes and a Vision." *New York Times*. Published July 19. www.nytimes.com/2015/07/19 /business/at-zappos-selling-shoes-and-a-vision.html.

Gesquire, L. R., N. H. Learn, M. C. Simao, P. O. Onyango, S. C. Alberts, and J. Altmann. 2011. "Life at the Top: Rank and Stress in Wild Male Baboons." *Science* 333 (6040): 357–60.

Gevinson, T. 2013. "I Want It to Be Worth It: An Interview with Emma Watson." *Rookie Magazine*. Published May 27. www .rookiemag.com/2013/05/emma-watson-interview.

Gladwell, M. 2010. "Speaking Is Not an Act of Extroversion." *Guardian*. Published June 21. www.theguardian.com/books /video/2010/jun/21/malcolm-gladwell.

Godsey, M. 2015. "When Schools Overlook Introverts." *Atlantic*. Published September 28. www.theatlantic.com/education /archive/2015/09/introverts-at-school-overlook/407467/.

Grant, A. 2014. "5 Myths About Introverts and Extraverts at Work." *Huffington Post*. Published February 19. www.huffingtonpost .com/adam-grant/5-myths-about-introverts_b_4814390.html.

Grant, A., F. Gino, and D. Hofmann. 2011. "Reversing the Extra-verted Leadership Advantage: The Role of Employee Proactiv-ity." *Academy of Management Journal* 54 (3): 528–50.

Grijalva, E., P. Harms, D. Newman, B. Gaddis, and R. C. Fraley. 2015. "Narcissism and Leadership: A Meta-Analytic Review of

Linear and Nonlinear Relationships." *Personnel Psychology* 68 (1): 1–47.

Guerber, H. A. 2012. *The Myths of Greece and Rome*. North Chelmsford, MA: Courier Corporation.

Hamilton, L. M., and C. M. Knoche. 2007. "Modesty in Leadership: A Study of the Level Five Leader." *International Journal of Servant Leadership* 3 (9): 139–76.

Hareli, S., and B. Weiner. 2000. "Accounts for Success as Determinants of Perceived Arrogance and Modesty." *Motivation and Emotion* 24 (3): 215–36.

Hoekstra, E., A. Bell, and S. R. Peterson. 2008. "Humility in Leadership: Abandoning the Pursuit of Unattainable Perfection." In *Executive Ethics: Ethical Dilemmas and Challenges for the C-Suite*, edited by S. A. Quatro and R. R. Sims, 79–96. Greenwich, CT: Information Age Publishing.

Hogan, R., R. Raskin, and D. Fazzini. 1990. "The Dark Side of Charisma." In *Measures of Leadership*, edited by K. E. Clark and M. B. Clark, 343–54. West Orange, NJ: Leadership Library of America.

Johnson, M., W. Rowatt, and L. Petrini. 2011. "A New Trait on the Market: Honesty-Humility as a Unique Predictor of Job Performance Ratings." *Personality and Individual Differences* 50 (6): 857–62.

Jones, D. 2006. "Not All Successful CEOs Are Extroverts." *USA Today*. Published June 7. http://usatoday30.usatoday.com /money/companies/management/2006-06-06-shy-ceo-usat_x .htm.

Judge, T., J. LePine, and B. L. Rich. 2006. "Loving Yourself Abundantly: Relationship of the Narcissistic Personality to Self and Other Perceptions of Workplace Deviance, Leadership, and Task and Contextual Performance." *Journal of Applied Psychology* 91 (4): 762–76.

Jung, C. G. 1921. *Psychological Types*. Vol. 6. Edited and translated by G. Adler and R. F. C. Hall. Princeton, NJ: Princeton University Press.

Kim, L. 2015. "30 Surprising Facts About Billionaire Tycoon Larry Ellison." *Inc. Magazine*. Published April 14. www.inc.com/larry-kim /30-surprising-facts-about-billionaire-tycoon-larry-ellison.html.

Klein, K., B. C. Lim, J. Saltz, and D. Mayer. 2004. "How Do They Get There? An Examination of the Antecedents of Centrality in Team Networks." *Academy of Management Journal* 47 (6): 952–63.

Krausea, N., K. Pargament, P. Hill, and G. Ironsond. 2016. "Humility, Stressful Life Events, and Psychological Well-being: Findings from the Landmark Spirituality and Health Survey." *Journal of Positive Psychology* 11 (5): 1–12.

LaBouff, J., W. Rowatt, M. Johnson, J. A. Tsang, and G. Willerton. 2011. "Humble Persons Are More Helpful Than Less Humble Persons: Evidence from Three Studies." *Journal of Positive Psychology* 7 (1): 16–29.

Lamb, E. 2016. Phone interview. February 18.

Lublin, J. S. 2015. "The Case for Humble Executives." *Wall Street Journal*. Published October 20. www.wsj.com/articles /the-case-for-humble-executives-1445385076.

Maccoby, M. 2004. "Narcissistic Leaders: The Incredible Pros, the Inevitable Cons." *Harvard Business Review*. Published January. https://hbr.org/2004/01/narcissistic-leaders -the-incredible-pros-the-inevitable-cons.

MacIntyre, P., and K. Thivierge. 1995. "The Effects of Speaker Personality on Anticipated Reactions to Public Speaking." *Communication Research Report* 12 (2): 125–33.

Martinuzzi, B. 2009. *The Leader as a Mensch: Become the Kind of Person Others Want to Follow*. San Francisco: Six Seconds Emotional Enterprise Press.

May, K. T. 2014. "How to Teach a Young Introvert." *TED*. Published September 2. http://ideas.ted.com/how-to-teach-a-young-introvert/.

Myers-Briggs Foundation. 2017. "MBTI Basics." Accessed March 7. www.myersbriggs.org/my-mbti-personality-type/mbti-basics/.

Nevicka, B., M. Baas, and F. Ten Velden. 2016. "The Bright Side of Threatened Narcissism: Improved Performance Following Ego Threat." *Journal of Personality* 84 (6): 809–23.

Nielsen, R., J. A. Marrone, and H. S. Ferraro. 2013. *Leading with Humility*. London: Routledge.

Ong, C. W., R. Roberts, C. Arthur, T. Woodman, and S. Akehurst. 2015. "The Leader Ship Is Sinking: A Temporal Investigation of Narcissistic Leadership." *Journal of Personality* 84 (12): 237–47.

O'Reilly, C., III, B. Doerr, D. Caldwell, and J. Chatman. 2014. "Narcissistic CEOs and Executive Compensation." *The Leadership Quarterly* 25 (2): 218–31.

Ou, A., A. Tsui, A. Kinicki, D. Waldman, Z. Xiao, and L. Song. 2014. "Humble Chief Executive Officers' Connections to Top Management Team Integration and Middle Managers' Responses." *Administrative Science Quarterly* 59 (1): 34–72.

Owens, B., and D. Hekman. 2016. "How Does Leader Humility Influence Team Performance? Exploring the Mechanisms of Contagion and Collective Promotion Focus." *Academy of Management Journal* 59 (3): 1088–111.

Owens, B., M. Johnson, and T. Mitchell. 2013. "Expressed Humility in Organizations: Implications for Performance, Teams, and Leadership." *Organization Science* 24 (5): 1517–38.

Owens, B. P., A. S. Wallace, and D. A. Waldman. 2015. "Leader Narcissism and Follower Outcomes: The Counterbalancing Effect of Leader Humility." *Journal of Applied Psychology* 100 (4): 1203–13.

Patel, P., and D. Cooper. 2014. "The Harder They Fall, the Faster They Rise: Approach and Avoidance Focus in Narcissistic CEOs." *Strategic Management Journal* 35 (10): 1528–40.

Paulhus, D. L. 1998. "Interpersonal and Intrapsychic Adaptiveness of Trait Self-enhancement: A Mixed Blessing?" *Journal of Personality and Social Psychology* 74 (5): 1197–208.

Pavot, W., E. Diener, and F. Fujita. 1990. "Extraversion and Happiness." *Personality and Individual Differences* 11 (12): 1299–306.

Pfeffer, J. 2015. *Leadership BS: Fixing Workplaces and Careers One Truth at a Time.* New York: HarperCollins.

Prime, J., and E. Salib. 2014a. *Inclusive Leadership: The View From Six Countries.* Catalyst. Accessed March 7. www.catalyst.org /system/files/inclusive_leadership_the_view_from_six _countries_0.pdf.

———. 2014b. "The Best Leaders Are Humble Leaders." *Harvard Business Review.* Published May 12. https://hbr.org/2014/05 /the-best-leaders-are-humble-leaders.

Raskin, R., and H. Terry. 1988. "A Principal-Components Analysis of the Narcissistic Personality Inventory and Further Evidence of Its Construct Validity." *Journal of Personality and Social Psychology* 54 (5): 890–902.

Shamir, B., R. J. House, and M. B. Arthur. 1993. "The Motivational Effects of Charismatic Leadership: A Self-concept Based Theory." *Organization Science* 4 (4): 577–94.

Stelmack, R. 2004. *On the Psychobiology of Personality: Essays in Honor of Marvin Zuckerman.* New York: Elsevier.

Susman, W. 1984. *Culture as History: The Transformation of American Society in the Twentieth Century.* New York: Pantheon Books.

Totten, K. 2015. "Living Small: At Downtown's Airstream Park, Home Is Where the Experiment Is." *Las Vegas Weekly.* Published February 5. http://lasvegasweekly.com/news/2015/feb/05 /airstream-park-experiment-living-small-hsieh-downt/.

Vera, D., and A. Rodriguez-Lopez. 2004. "Strategic Virtues: Humility as a Source of Competitive Advantage." *Organizational Dynamics* 33 (4): 393–408.

Waldman, D. A., and D. E. Bowen. 2016. "Learning to Be a Paradox-Savvy Leader." *Academy of Management Perspectives* 30 (3): 316–27.

Wales, W. J., P. Patel, and G. T. Lumpkin. 2013. "In Pursuit of Greatness: CEO Narcissism, Entrepreneurial Orientation, and Firm Performance Variance." *Journal of Management Studies* 50 (6): 1041–69.

Williams, C. 2011. *Management*, 6th ed. Mason, OH: South-Western Cengage Learning.

Wilson, M. 2003. *The Difference Between God and Larry Ellison: Inside Oracle Corporation.* New York: HarperCollins.

Zappos. 2010. "The Zappos Core Values." *Inc.* Published March 16. www.inc.com/inc-advisor/zappos-managin-people-zappos-core-values.html.

CHAPTER 3

Compassion

1

I<small>F YOU'RE UNDER</small> 35, you've probably never heard of Al Dunlap. Dunlap served, among other roles, as the CEO of Sunbeam, a company that made barbecues, blenders, and other home appliances in the 1990s. He was cruel, egotistical, and ill-tempered. He wrote a self-promoting book titled *Mean Business*. He earned the nicknames "Chainsaw Al" and "Rambo in Pinstripes," which he took as compliments. "You're not in business to be liked. Neither am I. We're here to succeed. If you want a friend, get a dog. I'm not taking any chances, I've got two dogs," he once said (Clikeman 2013, 205).

In the book *Chainsaw*, author John Byrne (2003) describes the first corporate meeting in the penthouse boardroom at Sunbeam headquarters in Fort Lauderdale, Florida, shortly after Dunlap had taken over as CEO in 1996.

> At precisely 9 A.M., on this Monday, July 22, Albert J. Dunlap marched into the room without introduction, without issuing a single greeting to any of the anxious men around the table. He looked exactly as he appeared in many of the photographs that accompanied the various articles the men had read that weekend. He wore his pinstripes like a military uniform, meticulously pressed, without a single

wrinkle or a stray thread, and perfectly fitted to his stocky frame. A white handkerchief peeked out of the chest pocket on his dark blue suit jacket. On his left hand, he sported a chunky West Point class ring above his gold wedding band.

The silver-haired Dunlap also wore a severe look on his face. His hard blue eyes, hidden by dark glasses, canvassed the room, fixing on each one of them. Only Spencer J. Volk, the baritone-voiced international president, was missing. Just moments before Dunlap's entrance, he had gone out to the men's room. And when he returned, no more than a minute past the appointed start time, Dunlap attacked him with vigor.

"Who are you?" he shouted as the man gingerly tiptoed to his seat.

"I'm Spencer Volk, sir. I'm head of international business," he said in a voice as smooth as a network television anchor's.

"Why are you late?" barked Dunlap.

"I was in the men's room," Volk nearly whispered.

"When I say we have a meeting at 9 o'clock," bellowed Dunlap, "it starts at 9! Gentlemen, look at your watches. Your lives will never be the same from this moment onward."

Like George C. Scott in the movie Patton, Dunlap began by delivering a spellbinding, if sometimes disjointed, monologue on himself and the company.

"The old Sunbeam is over today!" he proclaimed. "Let's get one thing clear: By God, I'm not Schipke. And I'm not Kazarian," he said, referring to the company's two previous chief executives, Roger Schipke and Paul Kazarian.

"You guys are responsible for the demise of Sunbeam!" Dunlap roared, tossing his glasses onto the table. "You are the ones who have played this political, bullshit game with Michael Price and Michael Steinhardt. You are the guys responsible for this crap, and I'm here to tell you that things have changed. The old Sunbeam is over today. It's over!"

Glaring fiercely, Dunlap kept repeating the phrase, again and again, saliva spattering from his lips. His chest was puffed out and his face flushed a bright red. The men stared in silence, incredulous at this outrageous performance, almost expecting Dunlap, like Patton, to slap someone out of frustration. Dunlap's bluster and mad grin, his oversized gleaming teeth too big for his face, seemed to fill the room. (Byrne 2003, 2–3)

Al Dunlap's behavior on that day set the tone for the rest of his reign at Sunbeam—he consistently used fear tactics and intimidation in dealing with his team and employees. But he was very good at what he did, which was turning failing companies into profitable enterprises. In 1994, when he took over Scott Paper (a company that makes sanitary tissue products), he tripled the company's market value in 20 months. Then he crafted a deal in which he sold it to Kimberly-Clark, earning the shareholders $6 billion. At Sunbeam, he propelled the share price from $12.25 to $52.25 in under two years.

While most people generally feared his brutality, many secretly admired his seemingly effective, no-nonsense style. In a 1996 letter to the editor of the *New York Times*, David Borsani, president of an appliance service agency, wrote: "I believe Al Dunlap . . . is one tough character who sets standards and expects people to meet those standards. He does not tolerate people who fill space unless they provide value. . . . Businesses are like houses: they eventually fill up with objects that contribute little to life but seem to be part of the landscape. Al Dunlap is very good at seeing life without the fluff" (Borsani 1996). When you can transform companies and make millions for your shareholders, very few will question the way you behave or how you treat others. For Al Dunlap, compassion and caring for his employees and fellow executives was irrelevant.

The word *compassion* comes from the Latin word *compati*: *com* means "together" and *pati* means "to suffer." In essence, being compassionate relates to the ability to feel with someone else, to sense his pain and suffering. The Tibetan scholar Thupten Jinpa defines compassion "as a mental state endowed with a sense of concern for the suffering of others and aspiration to see that suffering relieved." He explains that compassion has three components: a cognitive component that says to the other "I understand you," an affective component that says "I feel for you," and a motivational component that says "I want to help you" (Tan 2010, 199). This formulation implies that different processes are taking place in our minds when we feel compassion. First we notice the suffering. Then we make sense of it without being overwhelmed by it, then become emotionally connected to it, then try to alleviate the suffering through our words or actions.

A deep, underlying relationship exists among compassion, happiness, and love. When we feel compassion for others, we choose to turn away from a superficial focus on our own happiness to sense the true emotion and conditions of others. "The English word compassion is used to translate the Sanskrit *Karuna*, which is etymologized as *suspending happiness*," writes Robert Thurman, professor of Indo-Tibetan Buddhist studies at Columbia University (Thurman 2004, ix). When we are compassionate, we put our happiness on hold and focus on others' happiness, which requires us to have a true love for those others in the first place. Given that suffering and pain aren't obvious in the workplace, let's explore the relevance of compassion in the relationships that leaders have with their followers. Putting aside the Al Dunlap example, a large number of books and articles have made the case that compassion and empathy do have a place in leaders' feelings and actions.

Daniel Goleman, the emotional intelligence guru (a concept we'll discuss in depth in chapter 8), argues for the importance of empathy in leadership. He maintains that empathy is one of five skills that enable leaders to maximize their own potential and their followers' performance—the other four being self-awareness, self-regulation, motivation, and social skills. In the leadership context, empathy is the ability to understand the emotional makeup of other people and to treat them according to their emotional reactions. Goleman explains that "empathy doesn't mean a kind of 'I'm OK, you're OK' mushiness," nor does it mean to adopt other people's emotions as our own. Rather, "empathy means thoughtfully considering employees' feelings—along with other factors—in the process of making intelligent decisions" (Goleman 2004a). Therefore, an empathetic leader is in tune with employees' emotions, and he attracts, develops, and retains talent based on his deep understanding of others and their differences.

Goleman gives the real example of two division managers working in a large brokerage company that was merging with another company. As often happens in these cases, the merger resulted in many redundant jobs in some divisions. The first manager, too worried about his own fate, gathered his employees and gave them an insensitive and gloomy speech detailing the number of people who would be fired. The second manager, more empathetic in nature, was honest about his own worries and confusion but promised to treat his employees fairly and keep them informed of any changes. In the first division, many employees were demoralized and decided to leave, thus resulting in its ultimate demise. In contrast, employees in the second division felt that their manager intuitively related to them and acknowledged their fears. The best of them stayed, the division remained productive, and the manager emerged as a strong leader (Goleman 2004a).

In his remarkable book *Leaders Eat Last*, best-selling author and visionary thinker Simon Sinek (2014) relates a conversation he had with a lieutenant general from the Marine Corps. Sinek was wondering how Marines come to trust each other with their lives. The official attributed this tight-knit environment to empathetic leaders. He asked Sinek to go to any Marine Corps mess hall and watch the troops line up for their meal. Sinek observed that the most junior individuals ate first, and the leaders waited for everyone to finish before they served themselves. Sinek argues that empathy—the ability to recognize and share others' feelings—is the essence of leadership. He explains that empathy basically boils down to simple words when you notice something different about an employee: "Is everything OK?" It's also about little, everyday gestures that put the well-being of others first and that have a compounding and reciprocal effect on leader–follower relationships. While admitting that his vision of leadership is a bit idealistic, Sinek notes that "great leaders truly care about those they are privileged to lead and understand that the true cost of the leadership privilege comes at the expense of self-interest" (Sinek 2014, xiii).

Richard Boyatzis, professor at Case Western Reserve University, and Annie McKee, the cochair of the Teleos Leadership Institute, have advanced a related concept, *resonant leadership*. Resonant leaders use emotional and social intelligence skills to renew themselves, create positive relationships, and foster a healthy, vibrant environment to engage others in working toward a common goal. They do this through mindfulness, hope, and compassion. Boyatzis and McKee explain that "when experiencing compassion, a person does not assume or expect reciprocity or equal exchange. Compassion means giving selflessly" (Boyatzis and McKee 2005, 179). This understanding of compassion goes beyond the definition discussed earlier, which links compassion with caring for others who are in pain. In this sense, compassion is about reaching out and helping others regardless of whether their condition is based on suffering. Boyatzis and McKee's approach to compassion seems to be especially well-suited to the workplace: In most organizations, there is no real pain or suffering to be alleviated. Rather, compassionate leaders can help others achieve their goals and reach their full potential.

This thinking lines up well with the work of Geoff Aigner, the director of Social Leadership Australia. Aigner and his team use the term *social leadership* to reinforce the idea that leadership is about working for and with others (Aigner 2010). They believe that leadership is a social experience that involves other people and understanding who they are. For Aigner, part of the role of a leader is practicing compassion, transcending egos, and bringing happiness and love to employees' jobs and lives.

Google, one of the most sought-after workplaces in the United States, adheres to similar principles, with Chade-Meng Tan leading the way. Tan, or "Meng" to the people who know him, calls himself Google's "Jolly good fellow." He was one of the company's earliest engineers. Among many other achievements, he helped build Google's first mobile search service and headed the Google quality assurance team. In his recent book *Search Inside Yourself*, he argues that "the most compelling benefit of compassion in the context of work is that compassion creates highly effective leaders" (Tan 2010, 109). Similar to Jim Collins's conclusions in *Good to Great*, Tan suggests that the most effective leaders are those who combine compassion and humility with ambition, all for the greater good— that is, humbitious leaders. The affective and cognitive components of compassion tone down the excessive self-obsession of the leader, and therefore engender humility, whereas the motivational aspect of compassion creates an ambition to foster the greater good.

3

Despite those ideas, Al Dunlap's leadership style has been accepted in many organizations for a long time. Jerks are generally tolerated and sometimes celebrated by boards of trustees if they can get the job done. Scary leaders can push their followers to overperform via nasty stares, put-downs, and bullying. Some people would argue that Al Dunlap and other abrasive managers act the way leaders are supposed to act. They believe that lack of concern for other people's feelings isn't a defect, but rather something that is built into human nature, and that compassion and empathy are signs of weakness. Leaders are supposed to get results, and when they start caring about others' feelings, they may get distracted from their goals. Also, showing employees that you care about them may encourage them to think less of you and to try to take advantage of you.

The evidence shows that many historical and modern thinkers and philosophers advanced these ideas. For example, eighteenth-century German philosopher Immanuel Kant writes, "A feeling of sympathy is beautiful and amiable, for it shows a charitable interest in the lot of other men. . . . But this good-natured passion is nevertheless weak and always blind" (Keltner 2009, 227).

Friedrich Nietzsche, another brilliant German philosopher, alleges that humans are egocentric and self-seeking by nature, and that no true altruistic deeds exist. He concedes that some people perform kind deeds for others, which may make them appear considerate, caring, and selfless. But their innate intentions are always self-absorbed (Keltner 2009). Thomas Henry Huxley, the nineteenth-century British biologist and one of Charles Darwin's greatest students, argues that evolution didn't produce a biologically based capacity to care among humans. He is convinced that compassion and empathy aren't human states but rather cultural creations that are constructed within norms and religious commandments (Keltner 2009).

The more recent ideas of Ayn Rand, the influential Russian-American philosopher and novelist, are worth examining because they remain so popular in the United States long after her death in 1982. Rand is so admired that in one poll by the Library of Congress, readers ranked her novel *Atlas Shrugged* second only to the Bible in terms of books that have influenced them the most. Her books still sell more than half a million copies a year, and many have been made into movies. Rand established a doctrine called *objectivism* in which logic was central. She believed that emotion has no place in any human endeavor. In one of her novels, she praises the protagonist: "He does not understand, because he has no organ for understanding, the necessity, meaning, or importance of other people" (Burns 2011, 25). In another book she argues that people must reject the morality of altruism for the survival of society (Rand 1982). Numerous CEOs and politicians still swear by Rand's ideas. John Allison, the president and CEO of the Cato Institute and the previous chairman and CEO of BB&T Corporation, is a major contributor to the Ayn Rand Institute. He has made *Atlas Shrugged* required reading for all of his senior executives. When he was at BB&T, the company donated millions of dollars to colleges and universities on the condition that Rand's books and philosophy be extensively taught (Luskin and Greta 2013).

Rand's and others' ideas soon found their way into corporate America. In 1976, psychoanalyst Michael Maccoby interviewed 250 employees, ranging from chief executives to lower-level managers, in 12 well-known companies, for a study of what motivates them. In many of the interviews, managers describe how developing or employing qualities such as compassion or empathy would keep them from meeting corporate goals. "One [manager] was flabbergasted by the very idea of sensing his subordinates' feelings, of developing a heart that listens," Maccoby writes. He quotes another manager: "If I let myself feel their problems, I'd never get anything done. It would be impossible to deal with the people" (Maccoby 1976, 102). Many others believed that they needed to be emotionally detached from their employees in order to make decisions that might put these employees out of work, such as building new factories or changing technology. These philosophers, authors, and managers argue that human beings are naturally self-centered, and that those who show compassion and care for others tend to be weaker and less successful, especially in the workplace.

4

The fact that these reviews aren't universally shared may be unsurprising. But you would be shocked to know which ancient and recent thinkers and philosophers land in the camp that argues that compassion is a natural human trait. One of them is Charles Darwin—the same Darwin that came up with evolutionary theory. Eleven years before his death, Darwin published a little-known book called *The*

Descent of Man, in which he writes that concern for the welfare of others is shared among humans and animals.

One day, Darwin met a keeper at the Zoological Gardens in London. The keeper had deep wounds on his neck and relayed that a baboon had attacked him. What really caught Darwin's attention was that the keeper had a little American monkey that was very attached to him but that was very scared of the baboon. When the baboon attacked the keeper, the little monkey started screaming and biting the large animal. He managed to distract the baboon long enough for the keeper to escape. Darwin reflects on this incident: "Nevertheless, many a civilized man who never before risked his life for another, but full of courage and sympathy, has disregarded the instinct of self-preservation and plunged at once into a torrent to save a drowning man, though a stranger. In this case man is impelled by the same instinctive motive, which made the heroic little American monkey . . . save his keeper by attacking the great and dreadful baboon" (Ekman 2010). Contrary to the view of human nature as competitive and selfish that some have attributed to his theories, Darwin makes a strong case that sympathy is the strongest human instinct. Maybe what Darwin really means is that survival isn't for the fittest, but rather for the kindest.

Another example is that of Adam Smith, the father of economics. Smith is most famous for the concept of the "invisible hand of the market," which refers to the unobservable market forces that help the supply and demand of goods and services in a free market to reach equilibrium. Smith posits that an economy can work well in a free market scenario in which everyone works for her own interest. But in a less known publication, he advances the idea that the pursuit of self-interest should be tempered by "fellow feeling." He explains that "how selfish so ever man may be supposed, there are evidently some principles in his nature, which interest him in the fortune of others, and render their happiness necessary to him, though he derives nothing from it except the pleasure of seeing it" (de Waal 2009, 2). Even Smith, the most rational of economists, recognizes the importance of caring for others. It's clear that there are opposing views on whether human beings are naturally selfish or caring. So let's go beyond the opinions and explore the insights offered by modern science.

5

In the last few years, advances in behavioral and neurological studies have revealed some fascinating facts. Frans de Waal is a Dutch-born biologist and one of the world's best-known primatologists. De Waal has studied capuchin monkeys for years. These animals are very smart and cooperate well, both with each other and with humans, which makes them ideal for behavioral experiments. In one such experiment, de Waal and his team tested whether the capuchins recognize the needs of others, a quality seen as empathetic. The monkeys were offered food and were given the choice to share some of their food with another monkey. In the first situation, the other monkey had just eaten, whereas in the second situation, the other monkey had not eaten. Repeatedly, the monkeys that were offered the food shared more with monkeys who had no food than with ones whom they had just seen eating. This experiment suggests that a monkey's willingness to share food with another monkey depends on whether it has seen it eat or not (de Waal 2009).

In another experiment, de Waal and his team tested monkeys' interest in other monkeys' welfare. Two different-colored tokens were placed in front of a pair of monkeys. If a monkey picked one type of token (the "prosocial" token) and brought it to the scientist, both monkeys received apple pieces. If the monkey picked the other color (the "selfish" token) and brought it to the scientist, only that monkey received a piece of an apple and the other monkey received nothing. Because the monkey picking the token was rewarded regardless of which token it picked, the only difference was what the other monkey received. Over and over, the monkeys picked the prosocial token over the selfish token, which implies that monkeys, which are biologically very close to humans, have an innate capacity for empathy and compassion (de Waal 2009).

Recent scientific discoveries have even suggested that the capacity to care for others can be observed at the physiological level. In the human body, the vagus nerve originates in the top of the spinal cord and is threaded throughout the body, sending a variety of signals to the organs and transferring signals back to the brain. This nerve is responsible for the function and regulation of several bodily systems, such as the cardiovascular and digestive systems. A number of physiological psychologists have lately made the case that the vagus nerve is the compassion nerve.

University of California, Berkeley, psychology professor Dacher Keltner describes an experiment in which two sets of participants were shown different pictures. The first set was shown pictures that were meant to induce compassion: images of malnourished children, suffering during wartime, and infants in distress. The second set was shown pictures that induced pride: Because the participants were Berkeley undergraduates, the images included campus landmarks; images of sporting events; and Oski the bear, the university's beloved mascot. As the participants viewed the images, activity in their vagus nerves was measured with electrodes attached to their chests. The results showed that brief exposure to images inducing compassion triggered activation of the vagus nerve more than exposure to images inducing pride (Keltner 2009).

The second part of the experiment involved asking the same participants how "similar" they felt to 20 other diverse groups. Those groups included Democrats, Republicans, saints, small children, convicted felons, terrorists, the homeless, the elderly, farmers, and Stanford University students, among others. The participants who felt compassion reported feeling similar to a broader group of people, and to more vulnerable groups such as the homeless, the ill, and the elderly, than those who had felt pride. Keltner concludes, "The kindness . . . [that makes up] healthy communities [is] rooted in a bundle of nerves that has been producing caretaking behavior in more than 100 million years of mammalian evolution. And the lives of individuals with highly active vagus nerves add yet another chapter to the story of how we are wired to be good" (Keltner 2009, 240). More research is needed to understand exactly how the vagus nerve is related to compassion, but this study suggests that the capacity to care for others is biological.

Another way to understand this notion is to study how humans react in a biological way to watching others experience pain. When a human being is given a painful stimulus, a part of his brain called the *pain matrix* lights up. In a set of experiments performed by German neuroscientist Tania Singer, people observed a loved one receiving a painful stimulus. The surprising finding was that the same pain matrix lit up in their brains. Therefore, in a very real way, people can experience the suffering of others even when they aren't receiving the same sensory input themselves (Singer and Bolz 2013).

6

How do we make sense of these findings in the context of insensitive and cruel leaders? Are such leaders ignoring their hardwired, compassionate selves when they engage in nasty, intimidating behaviors? When Al Dunlap insulted other executives or laid off hundreds of employees as part of his turnarounds, he clearly chose not to employ compassion. In the book *Bad Leadership*, Harvard University researcher Barbara Kellerman qualifies Dunlap as the poster child for "callous leadership." She describes his style as "uncaring or unkind. Ignored or discounted are the needs, wants, and wishes of most members of the group or organization, especially subordinates" (Kellerman 2004, 120). Dunlap was indifferent to the well-being and happiness of his management team and employees. He exerted brutal pressure on them, made them work long and exhausting hours, intimidated them, and forced them to pass that intimidation down the line.

During his 22-month tenure as CEO of Scott Paper, he fired 11,000 employees without skipping a beat. That's 11,000 people with families, the majority of them having worked their entire lives at the company. When he later arrived at Sunbeam, he wanted to maintain his reputation. He told his associates, "I don't want people to think I've lost my touch. I want big numbers [of cuts]" (Kellerman 2004, 135). When he earned shareholders $100 million during those 22 months at Scott, the last thing on his mind was sharing his happiness with others. "Dunlap created a culture of misery, an environment of moral ambiguity, indifferent to everything except the stock price. He did not lead by intellect or by vision, but by fear and intimidation. . . . The pressure was beyond tough. It was barbarous," Kellerman reflects (Kellerman 2004, 135). I hope that by now you're starting to conclude that Al Dunlap is the exception, not the rule. In the next section, I'll present evidence that compassion and success in leadership are empirically related.

7

Gallup, the research and performance management consulting company, has been collecting data on leadership strengths for nearly 30 years. It has studied more than a million work teams, and it has conducted more than 20,000 interviews with leaders and more than 10,000 interviews with followers. In the noted book *Strengths Based Leadership*, author Tom Rath and leadership consultant Barry Conchie (2008) reveal some of the results of these interviews. According to the research, the most effective leaders understand their followers' needs and are invested in their followers' strengths. A leader with exceptional strength in this area is a developer of relationships, a good relater, and an includer of others. She is also characterized by empathy, harmony, connectedness, and positivity.

Rath and Conchie explain what it means to lead with empathy: "People strong in the empathy theme can sense the feelings of other people by imagining themselves in others' lives or situations" (Rath and Conchie 2008, 163). Those types of leaders build trust by helping "others articulate and frame complex emotions when they're faced with a worrisome situation" (Rath and Conchie 2008, 163). Their compassion comes from the fact that witnessing the happiness of others brings them pleasure. Therefore, they're "likely to be attuned to opportunities to highlight people's successes and positively reinforce their achievement" and sometimes "have the ability to understand what others are feeling before they've recognized it themselves" (Rath and Conchie 2008, 163). Empathy is important during hard times (as we saw in the merger example before) because it helps leaders demonstrate their concern, which can build loyalty and security. Moreover, empathetic leaders are typically chosen as confidantes or mentors by their followers. They encourage their employees by putting words to what they sense about aspirations and by coimagining dreams, which helps create hope in the organization.

The Gallup interviews with the followers aimed to answer the question, Who do people follow? The participants were asked to describe the leaders who have had the most positive influence on their lives and identified four basic follower needs: compassion, trust, stability, and hope. Rath and Conchie (2008, 85) expand on compassion: "Unfortunately, most leaders are hesitant to show genuine compassion for the people they lead, at least in the same way they would with a friend or family member. But the results of our studies suggest that it might be wise for these leaders to take a lesson from great managers, who clearly *do* care about each of their employees." So having compassionate and caring leaders is important, and followers seem to appreciate that. But compassion isn't just about warm, fuzzy feelings—years of evidence indicate that it can have a direct effect on organizational outcomes such as effectiveness, quality, and profitability.

In a separate study, more than 10 million people were asked to respond to the statement, "My supervisor, or someone at work, seems to care about me as a person." People who agreed with this statement were significantly more likely to stay with their organization, have more engaged customers, be substantially more productive, and generate more profitability for the organization (Rath and Conchie 2008).

Leadership experts Jim Kouzes and Barry Posner agree with this view. "For years, we've operated under the myth that leaders ought to be cool, aloof, and analytical; they ought to separate emotion from work. We're told that real leaders don't need love, affection, and friendship. 'It's not a popularity contest' is a phrase we've all heard often: 'I don't care if people like me. I just want them to respect me.' Nonsense," they write (Kouzes and Posner 2017). They argue that the best leaders care about how others feel and think, and that they want to be liked.

Research from the Center for Creative Leadership (2010), in which high-performing and low-performing managers were compared, also supports this view. Three interpersonal relationship factors were considered: inclusion, control, and affection. The results show that the only difference between the two groups was that top managers scored higher on affection than bottom ones. The highest-performing managers were more likely to show warmth and fondness toward others, got closer to their employees, and were more open to sharing their thoughts and feelings. Even in a no-nonsense environment such as the military, caring for others translates to higher performance. In one study, executive coach and organizational development consultant Wallace Bachman found that the most effective US Navy commanders are "more positive and outgoing, more emotionally expressive and dramatic, warmer and more sociable (including smiling more), friendlier and more democratic, more cooperative, more likable and 'fun to be with,' more appreciative and trustful, and even gentler than those that were merely average" (Goleman 2004b, 188). Therefore, clear evidence exists that compassionate leaders can be highly effective and can help produce positive outcomes in their organizations.

8

So far, I've discussed compassion and leadership in nonhealthcare sectors of the economy. Now we turn to healthcare. Healthcare is a natural place to discuss compassion—after all, hospitals and healthcare providers are in the business of compassion. Leadership competencies have been a focus in healthcare in the last decade. In that area, the work of management and search consultant Carson Dye and Rush University professor Andrew Garman is noteworthy. Based on inputs from board members, executives, search consultants, and executive coaches, Dye and Garman identify 16 leadership competencies that can be categorized into four traits: *well-cultivated self-awareness, compelling vision, masterful style of execution,* and *a real way with people*. They explain that having a "real way with people is listening like you mean it, giving feedback, mentoring others, developing teams, and energizing staff" (Dye and Garman 2006, xxiii). When leaders listen, provide feedback, and are involved in their employees' development and well-being, they're obviously exercising compassion.

Other work in healthcare shows that leadership dimensions can be divided into tangible and intangible factors. Healthcare consultant and leadership expert Tom Atchison argues that clinical and business processes (the "tangibles") account for only 35 percent of organizational performance, whereas deeper dimensions of leadership (the "intangibles") account for the other 65 percent (Atchison 2006). Based on his 22 years of experience, Atchison proposes that the intangible dimensions are trust, respect, pride, and joy. Trust takes times and is cultivated through meaningful interactions and listening. Respect is built on trust—it thrives in an environment in which performers are acknowledged for their good work. Pride is the result of meeting meaningful challenges. Trust, respect, and pride are needed to have joy, and Atchison argues that feeling joy at work is the highest level of performance that a leader can create in the organization.

The work of healthcare author and consultant Michael Frisina has touched on similar issues. He presents the concept of *influential leadership* and identifies three fundamental principles: self-awareness, collaboration, and connection (Frisina 2014). Frisina explains that connection is a strategy used by leaders to show that they care for and understand the needs of their employees. One of the true measures of a successful leader is whether her employees are willing to follow her in good times and bad. Frisina suggests that the factors that drive employees to follow their leaders are trust, compassion, stability, and hope. Influential leaders understand that people need to emotionally bond with them in order to connect with their work and perform, and therefore they intentionally form meaningful relations with those around them.

Along the same lines, employees in highly participative work climates demonstrate better customer service, commit fewer medication errors, are less burned out, and are less likely to leave the organization than employees in more authoritarian work climates. This result is outlined in a study conducted at the Spartanburg Regional Healthcare System in South Carolina, which examined the relationship between participative management and organizational outcomes. These findings tell us that open communication and shared decision making between managers and followers, which are related to compassion, can have a strong influence on employees' performance, emotions, and loyalty (Angermeiner et al. 2009). To gain an even deeper understanding of compassion in healthcare organizations, I set out to talk to some proven leaders.

9

In 1869, the Catholic bishop of Texas sent a call asking for help in caring for the sick, infirm, and orphaned on the Texas frontier. The Sisters of Charity of the Incarnate Word responded to the call and founded CHRISTUS Santa Rosa Hospital. Santa Rosa currently has five hospitals in its health system, with more than 1,000 beds and a number of specialty centers. Don Beeler was the president and CEO of CHRISTUS Santa Rosa Health System in San Antonio from 2003 to 2010. His career spanned 35 years of high-level leadership positions across several healthcare organizations.

When I called Don to ask him to talk about leadership issues, I suggested that we meet at a coffee shop. Instead, Don kindly invited me to his house. He joked, "It's more comfortable, and the coffee is free." When I arrived at his house in an old San Antonio, Texas, neighborhood on a rainy fall day, he was waiting for me in the driveway with his unmistakable wide smile. He explained that he had bought the house 40 years ago, when he was starting his career as an administrative resident at CHRISTUS Santa Rosa. He had returned to live there when he became its CEO. Coffee was already brewing in the pot. Don poured two cups and we made our way to a cozy living room decorated with horned frogs, in homage to his beloved Texas Christian University football team.

As we started talking, I brought up the topic of compassion in leadership. He immediately remarked that the topic resonates with him.

> It is probably a personality thing, but it is also a healthcare thing, which is more relational than any other industry. When I started my career as an administrative resident at Santa Rosa, my first mentor was a nun. She was the administrator and the chairman of the board. During board meetings, she made it a habit to serve coffee to everyone. I asked her, "Why do you do that? There are people from the dietary department who can do that." She said, "Those members of the board sitting around the table are giving from themselves and from their time to this organization; I want them to understand that we also serve them." For her, it was reciprocal, it was a small gesture, but it was the natural thing to do. I made observations about that, about how she was a servant leader. She wasn't wrapped up in her title. Of course, she did all the other things such as the rules and expectations to get things done. This has shaped how I look at the world. (Beeler 2014)

This leadership lesson has stayed with Don throughout his career. While his colleagues working in other places were focused on rules and policies, his emphasis was on the relational issues. He explains further, "In themselves, the relational issues won't produce any results, but with clear rules and expectations, they will" (Beeler 2014). As Don started climbing the executive ladder, he kept that in mind and practiced compassion and respect in the treatment of his people.

> If you want respect, you should respect the people and their careers. You demonstrate compassion to your employees as individuals. When I was working, I rarely socialized with people I worked with outside of work because I thought it might compromise the relationship with them. But there is a difference between being a buddy and a compassionate, sincere leader. I spent time with them not just in groups, but individually too, on a regular basis. I told them, "I am interested in your career." And I told them that if a good opportunity comes up for them to work somewhere else, I would help them. Of course I didn't want to lose my people, but I needed them to know that I cared about their careers. (Beeler 2014)

Don explains that compassion isn't about being "Mr. Nice Guy"—it's also important in getting results. He notes, "You have to clarify expectations and be honest: 'Hey, this is not going as well as I hoped, this is where we need to be, in terms of budget, satisfaction scores, costs, etc.' You have to be honest, but not mean or nasty. You have to respect the person, even if you are not happy with the behavior or the outcome" (Beeler 2014). Don clearly believes that showing compassion is an important aspect of being a leader, and he has produced outstanding results practicing this brand of leadership. During his tenure, CHRISTUS Santa Rosa was recognized as one of the top 5 percent of hospitals in the country for clinical excellence for seven straight years. Among other achievements, he helped build and open a new 150-bed hospital, successfully acquired another hospital, and formed four ambulatory surgery center joint ventures with physicians. Clearly, leaders in healthcare can be compassionate and effective at the same time.

10

Are Don Beeler's views shared by other people working in healthcare? In my survey, I asked employees, supervisors, directors, and executives to think about the one leader they have observed to be the most successful in terms of improving outcomes in the organization (e.g., quality, financial) and getting things done. Then I asked them to describe that leader by choosing five traits from a list. Being accountable topped the other traits, with 64 percent of the respondents choosing it to describe their successful leader. This characteristic was followed by being collaborative (54 percent), holding others accountable (48 percent), and being calm (40 percent). Compassion came in at fifth place, with 39 percent of the respondents picking it to describe a successful leader. The picture painted is that strong leadership, characterized by being accountable and holding others accountable, collaboration, calmness, and compassion, can lead to real success in healthcare organizations.

I also asked the same group to think about the leader who has had the most positive influence on their careers. Using the same list, the top two traits were being accountable (59 percent) and compassionate (52 percent), followed by being collaborative (50 percent) and calm (48 percent). When healthcare employees, managers, and executives of all levels think of a leader who has helped them along in their careers, they think of a leader who feels with them, who works well with them in a calm and assured way, and who is accountable for his actions. (See the appendix at the end of the book for the complete survey results.)

11

Back to Al Dunlap. As it turns out, the results that he produced for Sunbeam were short-lived. A few months after declaring victory, things took a turn for the worse. Between March and May of 1998, Sunbeam's stock dropped by 50 percent. The company was $2 billion in debt. It was discovered that Dunlap had used accounting tricks, such as moving up sales dates for consumer goods ahead of delivery, in an effort to advance quarterly sales numbers. He also lied to investors. At his last investors' meeting, he was challenged by 200 fuming shareholders over these practices. Dunlap confronted them angrily, placing his hand over one employee's mouth and yelling into the employee's ear, "You son of a bitch. If you want to come after me, I'll come after you twice as hard" (Fastenberg 2010). Shortly after, Dunlap was fired over the phone. Former employees "nearly danced" in the streets. In its June 18, 1998, edition, under the title "Al Dunlap: Exit Bad Guy," the *Economist* wrote, "To many Americans, June 15th was a day for rejoicing. After all, it isn't every day that a true villain is vanquished—especially one as irredeemable as Al Dunlap" (*Economist* 1998). A couple of years later, Sunbeam filed for bankruptcy. In 2010, *Time* named Dunlap one of the ten worst bosses in history (Fastenberg 2010).

What do we learn from the story of Al Dunlap? Sometimes, uncaring and abrasive leaders can get results by sheer intimidation and lack of consideration for others. But that seems to work only in the short term. Leaders who want to get long-term results and to leave a positive legacy are more successful when they include others while insisting on strict standards of accountability.

REFERENCES

Aigner, G. 2010. *Leadership Beyond Good Intentions: What It Takes to Really Make a Difference.* Crows Nest, Australia: Allen & Unwin.

Angermeiner, I., B. Denford, A. Boss, and W. Boss. 2009. "The Impact of Participative Management Perceptions on Customer Service, Medical Errors, Burnout and Turnover Intentions." *Journal of Healthcare Management* 54 (2): 127–40.

Atchison, T. 2006. *Leadership's Deeper Dimensions: Building Blocks to Superior Performance.* Chicago: Health Administration Press.

Beeler, D. 2014. Personal interview. November 5.

Borsani, D. 1996. "In Praise of Al Dunlap." *New York Times.* Published December 29. www.nytimes.com/1996/12/29 /business/l-in-praise-of-al-dunlap-937827.html.

Boyatzis, R., and A. McKee. 2005. *Resonant Leadership.* Boston: Harvard Business School Press.

Burns, J. 2011. *Goddess of the Market: Ayn Rand and the American Right.* New York: Oxford University Press.

Byrne, J. 2003. *Chainsaw: The Notorious Career of Al Dunlap in the Era of Profit-at-Any-Price.* New York: HarperCollins.

Center for Creative Leadership. 2010. *Addressing the Leadership Gap in Healthcare: What's Needed When It Comes to Leader Talent?* Published June. www.ccl.org/wp-content/uploads/2015/04 /addressingLeadershipGapHealthcare.pdf.

Clikeman, P. 2013. *Called to Account: Financial Frauds That Shaped the Accounting Profession.* New York: Routledge.

Dye, C., and A. Garman. 2006. *Exceptional Leadership: 16 Critical Competencies for Healthcare Executives.* Chicago: Health Administration Press.

Economist. 1998. "Al Dunlap: Exit Bad Guy." Published June 18. www.economist.com/node/136843.

Ekman, P. 2010. "Survival of the Kindest." *Mindful.* Published December 23. www.mindful.org/cooperate/.

Fastenberg, D. 2010. "Workplace Users and Abusers: Al Dunlap." *Time.* http://content.time.com/time/specials/packages /article/0,28804,2025898_2025900_2026107,00.html.

Frisina, M. 2014. *Influential Leadership: Change Your Behavior, Change Your Organization, Change Healthcare.* Chicago: Health Administration Press.

Goleman, D. 2004a. "What Makes a Leader?" *Harvard Business Review.* Published January. https://hbr.org/2004/01/what -makes-a-leader.

————. 2004b. *Working with Emotional Intelligence*. New York: Bantam Dell.

Kellerman, B. 2004. *Bad Leadership: What It Is, How It Happens, Why It Matters*. Boston: Harvard Business School Press.

Keltner, D. 2009. *Born to Be Good: The Science of a Meaningful Life*. New York: W. W. Norton & Company, Inc.

Kouzes, J. M., and B. Posner. 2017. "A Secret Revealed." Accessed March 9. www.leadershipchallenge.com/resource/encouraging-the-heart-a-secret-revealed.aspx.

Luskin, D. L., and A. Greta. 2013. "Business Hero John Allison: BB&T—The Bank That Atlas Built." *Capitalism Magazine*. Published April 25. http://capitalismmagazine.com/2013/04/business-hero-john-allison-bbt-the-bank-that-atlas-built/.

Maccoby, M. 1976. "The Corporate Climber Has to Find His Heart." *Fortune*, December, 98–110. www.maccoby.com/Articles/CorporateClimber.shtml.

Rand, A. 1982. *Philosophy: Who Needs It*. Indianapolis: Bobbs-Merrill.

Rath, T., and B. Conchie. 2008. *Strengths Based Leadership: Great Leaders, Teams, and Why People Follow*. New York: Gallup Press.

Sinek, S. 2014. *Leaders Eat Last: Why Some Teams Pull Together and Others Don't*. New York: Penguin Group.

Singer, T., and M. Bolz. 2013. *Compassion: Bridging Science and Practice*. Munich, Germany: Max Planck Society.

Tan, C. 2010. *Search Inside Yourself: The Unexpected Path to Achieving Success, Happiness (and World Peace)*. New York: HarperOne.

Thurman, R. 2004. "Foreword." In *The Lost Art of Compassion: Discovering the Practice of Happiness in the Meeting of Buddhism and Psychology*, by Lorne Ladner, ix–xi. San Francisco: HarperSanFrancisco.

Waal, F. de. 2009. *The Age of Empathy: Nature's Lessons for a Kinder Society*. New York: Harmony Books.

CHAPTER 4

Kindness

1

In *Divergent*, the popular book series for young adults, teenagers take an aptitude test when they reach the age of 16. Based on their scores, they're divided into five factions: Abnegation, Dauntless, Erudite, Amity, and Candor. Abnegation, the selfless faction, represents those who kindly serve others while completely forgetting about themselves. They dress in baggy gray clothes and sit quietly, and they're pejoratively nicknamed "stiffs." The Abnegation manifesto explains how members of this faction view themselves and the world:

> I will be my undoing if I become my obsession.
> I will forget the ones I love if I do not serve them.
> I will war with others if I refuse to see them.
> Therefore I choose to turn away from my reflection,
> To rely not on myself
> But on my brothers and sisters,
> To project always outward
> Until I disappear. (Roth 2017)

Dauntless is the brave faction, representing people who are fearless in the face of danger. They're loud and expressive; excel in fighting and physical skills; wear black clothing; and have tattoos, body piercings, and colored hair. The Erudite faction is characterized by great knowledge. Its members are curious and in constant pursuit of learning and technological advances—most wear glasses to give the appearance of intelligence. The last two factions are Amity, which seeks friendship and peaceful harmony, and Candor, which values sincerity and openness. Because they're deemed morally incorruptible, the Abnegations were originally considered the only faction capable of governing the city. However, because of their apparent submissive nature, other factions try to take advantage of them. The Dauntless members, for example, have little respect for the peacefulness and seeming cowardice of the Abnegation, while the Erudite members believe that the Abnegations are in fact selfish people who only provide for their own faction. Inevitably, the Dauntless and Erudite conspire to launch a genocide against the Abnegation, killing most of its members. *Divergent* is a dystopian series of novels that takes place in futuristic Chicago. But this representation of the kind as helpless and weak isn't uncommon in our society.

2

A significant and widespread suspicion of kindness and niceness is observable in our world today. (I will use the terms *kind* and *nice* interchangeably.) A kind person is sometimes perceived as someone who believes that his moral standards are perfect and that he is superior to others. He acts in a self-righteous way, is often condescending, and treats others with moral smugness. People are skeptical about those who put everyone's needs in front of their own. They believe that the main motivation for that behavior is to secretly exploit others and advance one's own agenda, and they can't understand how anyone could care so much about others without wanting anything in return.

Others consider kindness to be the lowest form of weakness; the kind are only kind because they don't have the guts to be anything else. In their 2009 book *On Kindness*, psychoanalyst Adam Phillips and historian Barbara Taylor note that "most people, as they grow up now, secretly believe that kindness is a virtue of losers" (Phillips and Taylor 2009, 9). A large number of us don't allow ourselves to be kind anymore. A coworker is struggling with a project with a tight deadline. A friend needs help with a presentation. We would like to help them, but we fear that we may be taken advantage of. Or that we won't have time to focus on our own priorities. Or that we may be jeopardizing our own chances for promotion or advancement. We don't want to be perceived as the office doormat. Because, deep down, some of us believe that human beings are bad and dangerous, that "we are deeply and fundamentally antagonistic to each other, that our motives are utterly self-seeking" (Phillips and Taylor 2009, 4).

These modern views originated from ideas advanced by the English philosopher Thomas Hobbes. In his 1651 book *Leviathan*, in which he established social contract theory, Hobbes dismisses Christian kindness as psychological absurdity (Hobbes 2010). He insists that men are selfish beasts who care for nothing but their own well-being. Many people today unknowingly adopt a Hobbesian perspective, convinced that self-interest is our ruling principle. As such, kindness is typically dismissed as weak and sentimental. After all, if you're too nice to people, they're likely to attack or insult you without fear of payback. As a kind person, you're perceived as nonconfrontational and even noncompetitive—and therefore, many may see you as unable to achieve success. As people sometimes say, "If you're a doormat, then you deserve to be stepped on."

3

Nowhere else is this view of niceness more prevalent than in the workplace. "Nice has an image problem. Nice gets no respect," write Linda Kaplan Thaler and Robin Koval, the CEO and president of the Kaplan Thaler Group, a successful advertising agency (Thaler and Koval 2006, 3). They suggest that nice people are considered "Pollyanna and passive, wimpy, and Milquetoast." When we think of nice people at work, we typically think of those who are constantly trying to please others; who value agreeableness over assertiveness; who treat others well by giving away their own personal power; who prioritize and cater to others' demands and wants over truthfulness and authenticity; and who constantly avoid and minimize disagreement, conflict, and discomfort. We also think of those who fail *because* of their niceness.

Linnaea Bohn, a former business executive, recalls a time early in her career when she was in management:

> When I worked in the corporate world, I didn't focus on a race to the top. I enjoyed the day-to-day work of running a product line, finding opportunities for new markets, and helping managers in other countries launch similar lines tailored to their markets. My approach was to be ethical in all aspects of the work, to have concern for the people I was working with to achieve results, and to share the credit appropriately. This was not the latest "management style," nor was it proven. The most senior managers saw the bottom line increase and gave me more responsibility and a promotion, while immediate supervisors discredited me since I was not like them. A transfer to Asia fortunately took me out of the quagmire of home office politics. I felt the freedom to continue managing in a way that was natural to me: to encourage my teams with kindness, cooperation, and credit while we increased market share and the bottom line. My staff felt safe and enjoyed their work. The division prospered. However, my immediate superior didn't value my approach. He viewed it as a sign of weakness that I was caring and thoughtful, and that I cooperated and shared with each colleague. Even though I had added millions to the bottom line, I lost my job, my career. (Bohn 2017)

Many people can relate to Bohn's situation and can remember a time when their niceness didn't fit with their organizational culture.

While this example shows an appropriate level of niceness went unappreciated by a certain boss, some people are overly nice, which gets in the way of their success. This tendency is sometimes referred to as the *nice guy syndrome.* According to Ross C. Edelman, Timothy R. Hiltabiddle, and Charles C. Manz (2008), this syndrome is characterized by a lack of self-awareness, which can lead nice people to be less effective, hindering their careers. Overly nice guys typically don't speak their minds because they fear being judged by others. Because they tend to be people pleasers, they're unable to set boundaries. They find it very hard to push back when someone makes an unreasonable request because they lack the ability to say no.

Overly nice people are nonconfrontational. This characteristic can be especially damaging when conflict remains unresolved, which can negatively affect productivity. Overly nice bosses, for instance, tend to be very lenient with their subordinates, often failing to hold them accountable because they're unable to have tough conversations and address poor performance. These shortcomings often lead to career failure. "Whether because of competitive pressure, a sense of unworthiness, a fear of sowing the seeds of future conflict, or concern over displacing others, many overly nice guys will shun the limelight and the winner's circle," explain Edelman, Hiltabiddle, and Manz (2008, 229). Excessive kindness can therefore get in the way of achievement. It can also be a major disadvantage in some leadership situations. Geoff Aigner, the Australian leadership expert that we met in chapter 3, explains that sometimes,

> out of kindness we don't tell someone how they are making things worse or not helping. Out of kindness we give people what they want in the short term to the detriment of the long term. Out of kindness we protect people form a difficult truth. . . . So we may not tell a colleague or subordinate they are not performing because they are fragile, come from a minority group or are difficult to deal with. We create a wide berth filled with cotton wool and ultimately,

unwittingly, ensure they can never get out of the spot they are in—we keep them stuck in their place. (Aigner 2011, 57)

Is it better to be nice with your staff members so they can like you or to be tough with them so they can respect you more and work harder? Emma Seppälä, the science director of Stanford University's Center for Compassion and Altruism Research and Education argues that most people believe the latter is best. In this traditional paradigm, leaders who are firm and a little distant are thought to instill respect and fear in their employees. They employ "a little dog-eat-dog, tough-it-out, sink-or-swim culture" that can keep people hungry and on their toes. They make it clear that they're in charge. As for leaders who seem as if they care a little too much, they might look too soft and be less respected, which may entice employees to work less hard (Seppälä 2014). In that sense, kindness can be seen as a stumbling block for leaders and is better left out of the workplace. But try telling that to the Mitchells.

4

In 1958, Ed and Norma Mitchell bought an 800-square-foot supply store in Westport, Connecticut, and opened a small clothing company. Their first inventory consisted of no more than three suits. Every day, Norma brought a pot of coffee to serve the customers and make them feel at home. Since those humble beginnings, the company has grown by leaps and bounds. Today, the Mitchells family of stores is a nationally renowned $60 million specialty clothing chain with locations in multiple cities. The main Mitchells store in Connecticut is more than 25,000 square feet, and the acquisition of other high-end stores with well-known brands in multiple locations has allowed the company to thrive.

The growth and success of the company is owed to an effective family business structure and sophisticated information technology.

But according to Ed and Norma, the secret sauce is a culture of niceness that they have cultivated and taught to their sons, nephews, and grandsons, all of whom work in the business. In this culture, employees have a pleaser mentality—they want to do nice things just to be nice. They engage one another as real people rather than as a responsibility of the job. In 2008, Jack Mitchell wrote a book called *Hug Your People*, in which he details how recognizing and encouraging his employees has helped him foster the business while keeping it humane. For him, to hug someone is to recognize a job well done, whether through an actual physical hug, a simple thank-you, or something more extravagant such as sending an employee on a trip (Mitchell 2008). Domenic Condoleo, the head tailor in Westport, was a soccer fanatic. So when the World Cup came to the United States in 1994, Ed paid for Domenic to go watch the games in New York, Boston, and Los Angeles!

Some skeptics may say that these touchy-feely practices can only work at a luxury clothing store operated by a close-knit family. But other examples of cultures of niceness come in all shapes and sizes. Most people have not heard of the SAS Institute, a business analytics software company based in North Carolina. SAS consistently ranks among *Fortune*'s hundred best places to work, primarily as a result of an uncommon philosophy based on treating employees kindly (as well as some outrageous perks). Leaders at SAS have made employee happiness one of their main goals. Legendary CEO Jim Goodnight explains the company's philosophy: "If you treat employees as if they make a difference to the company, they *will* make a difference" (Crowley 2013). For him, it's just common sense—treat people kindly, keep them challenged with interesting work, respect them, and appreciate their contributions, and they'll reward you with high performance. That philosophy guides Goodnight's thinking when he is selecting employees to be promoted to management—he doesn't look for people who are just competent and capable, he also looks for those who help and develop others. At SAS, leaders support their people and provide them with opportunities for growth and advancement. In other words, leaders are coaches, not dictators.

In addition to regular health and dental benefits, SAS employees enjoy some highly unusual perks that help them feel appreciated and be more productive. They have free access to a massive gymnasium featuring tennis and basketball courts, a weight room, and a heated pool. They also have a free on-site healthcare clinic, staffed by physicians, nutritionists, physical therapists, and psychologists. Parents can apply for deeply discounted on-campus Montessori childcare. They're encouraged to have lunch with their kids at one of the four restaurants managed by the company, where children can enjoy, among other treats, octopus-shaped hotdogs. Other services provided at the company include a hair stylist, a manicurist, and a massage therapist. Break rooms are stocked with free fresh fruit on Mondays and M&M candies on Wednesdays. Employees can leave the workplace at any time to take care of a family obligation or attend a child's event without having to ask for a supervisor's permission. They also enjoy unlimited sick days and flexible 36-hour weeks.

The evidence that the SAS approach works is clear: The company's revenues have increased for 33 consecutive years and its profit margins are consistently in the double digits. But most important, the average employee tenure is 10 years and turnover rate is 2 percent, in an industry where the average hovers around 20 percent. Every year, 40,000 applicants compete for 200 vacant positions at SAS. What other companies spend on selecting, recruiting, training, and replacing workers, SAS spends on perks and benefits—it's that simple. But that doesn't mean that the company hasn't faced challenges. In 2009, the recession forced almost every other software company to lay off large numbers of workers. Employees at SAS were justifiably worried that their company might follow suit. But Goodnight decided that it was time to address the anxiety: He held a global webcast for the company's 13,000 employees and announced that no one would be losing their jobs. He asked them to be cautious with spending and to help the company navigate these hard times. "By making it very clear that no one was going to be laid off," Goodnight said later, "suddenly we cut out huge amounts of chatter, concern, and worry—and people got back to work" (Tenney and Gordon 2014, 54). His employees rewarded his decision by producing even more breakthrough products while the competitors were slashing costs. SAS enjoyed record profits in 2009 (Brenoff 2013, 2014).

5

In 2012, Catholic Healthcare West, the fifth largest health system in the United States, announced that it was changing its name to Dignity Health. But this change affected more than just the logo. The leaders of the organization committed to changing the way they think of healthcare delivery. As the country's healthcare system was becoming more bureaucratic and impersonal, Dignity Health set out to bring compassion and kindness back into healthcare relationships and to unleash the "power of humanity."

The rebranding effort included extensive research and conversations with providers, employees, and patients. Providers and employees valued compassionate care, while patients wanted to be listened to and to be treated kindly. A national survey of patients commissioned by Dignity Health revealed some surprising findings. The respondents were asked to rank important considerations in choosing a healthcare provider. About 87 percent of them felt that kind treatment by a physician was more important than other factors, such as average wait time before appointments, distance from home, and the cost of care. The alarming news was that 64 percent had experienced unkind behavior in a healthcare setting, such as the failure of a caregiver to connect on a personal level, staff rudeness, or poor listening skills (AZBio 2017).

Fueled by these findings and by what they perceived as the general rise of incivility in society, Dignity Health executives launched an external and internal rebranding campaign called "Hello Humankindness" (one word, not a typo). Advertisements in major national newspapers featured a simple message: "Let's make kindness and humanity a part of every conversation and debate and policy decision.

Let's make it the absolute core that informs everything we say. And do" (Dignity Health 2013). A new hashtag, #hellohumankindness, was born online, and the organization issued the following manifesto:

Hello humankindness.
You hold the power to heal. To have a real impact on the health of the people around you. We all do. Which is why modern medicine is ripe for a change in perspective.

Because each of us is human. Our body, mind, and spirit is one and the same. So if our mind is calmer because we feel we are being taken care of by those around us, our body responds. Stress levels go down and we can heal faster.

This is the true power of humankindness. It's the effect we can have on one another when we reach out and help ease each other's pain. These beliefs are at the very core of our mission, and have been for over 100 years. Which is why we aim for nothing less than to inspire change in health care that leads to more empathy, listening, and respect. Alongside the latest in technology and medical breakthroughs, we can champion the healer in all of us. Not simply because it's nice, but because it's good for us.

And because it works. For all the negativity, disease, and toxicity in our lives, we have a very real and very powerful tool against it. We call it humankindness. And we believe it has the power to change not just health care, but the world in which we live.

Join us. For we are all caregivers at heart. (Dignity Health 2013)

This new approach was complemented by several strategic initiatives that were designed to create a patient experience aligned with the brand promise. The organization put into place kind human resource practices, programs that strengthen the connection between patients and providers, and services that empower patients and families and engage the broader community. To help spread the message internally among employees, managers were given brand development launch toolkits to help them in conversations about the new brand with employees and physicians. A new video titled *Unleashing the Healing Power of Humanity* became a staple at staff meetings, huddles, and town hall gatherings, while stories and ideas were shared in an online employee community.

"One of the most important tools we have to fight fear, uncertainty, and discomfort is perhaps also one of the most simple and inexpensive: kindness," writes Dr. Gary Greensweig, vice president and chief physician executive, in a 2014 article. "At Dignity Health, we are taking steps to develop a kinder community of care, both within our hospitals and throughout the areas we serve. Certainly this means employing basic courtesies in each of our patient interactions, including listening without interruption, maintaining steady eye contact, and paying careful attention to both the words and body language of our patients" (Greensweig 2014).

Intrigued by this positive message, I reached out to Gary to inquire about how these initiatives, primarily directed toward patients, have affected the way leaders treat their employees in the organization. Gary is a primary care physician who has held several leadership positions across the years while continuing to see patients. He joined the organization in 2012 as the new campaign was just starting—a "fascinating journey," as he describes it. He confessed that some of the leaders in the organization gravitated more quickly than others toward the new values. However, he credits the majority of executives and managers with walking the talk and spreading the message of humankindness to the staff by building kindness into their conversations; the requests they made; and the gestures that built relationships, trust, and familiarity among care teams. "Our president and CEO Lloyd Dean has been a major part of this advocacy and attended humankindness events in each of our service areas," he explains (Greensweig 2016).

The process has not been without challenges. Gary notes that there are "forces of nature" that can act as a deterrent to the campaign, such as challenges with reimbursement and the effects of cost reductions on staff. Despite these challenges, he believes that the efforts have been highly worthwhile, because the kindness message resonates so deeply with staff and clinicians. He tells the story of a meeting between executives and a group of doctors that historically have had a contentious relationship with one of the system hospitals. "As we started sharing with them the principles of the humankindness campaign, the leader of the physician group, a grown man in his sixties, started crying. 'This is what we have wanted from you all along,' he said" (Greensweig 2016). I finally asked Gary, a kind soul himself, what it meant for him as a leader to work in a system that prioritizes kindness as a value. "For me, it feels like I am at home in this environment. It is like something was missing and now I have found it" (Greensweig 2016).

6

What does it mean to be kind at work? And how does kindness affect leadership and performance? Being kind in the workplace is a consciously chosen approach to relationships that is founded on attempting to optimize outcomes for others and ourselves. Kind leaders regularly say "thank you" when their subordinates make a suggestion. They take time out of their busy day to check on employees and ask about their families. They welcome new employees with open arms and make sure the newcomers are comfortable and settled. They also train themselves to limit or eliminate nasty comments. Liz Jazwiec, author of *Eat THAT Cookie!* (2009), relates the story of a hospital nursing director who got tired of all the negative talk in her work area. At church one Sunday, she heard the pastor speak about the destructive effects of an untamed tongue. So she thought of a clever idea to address that issue with her employees: using tongue depressors. She held a meeting with the staff and expressed to them that she was not happy with the culture of unkindness that had developed in the unit. She showed them the tongue depressors, on which she had written scripture pertaining to negative words, and she asked each one of them to write their own messages on blank tongue depressors. She urged everyone, including herself, to stick the depressor in their mouth whenever they felt a negative comment coming to the surface. She also encouraged them to do the same whenever a coworker muttered a nasty comment. Gradually, the culture of the unit began to change and employee satisfaction scores increased dramatically.

Many people are starting to embrace the idea of niceness at work and suggest that it can even be a sign of strength. Thaler and Koval make an important point: "Let us be clear: Nice is not naive. Nice does not mean smiling blandly while others walk all over you. Nice does not mean being a doormat. In fact, we would argue that nice is the toughest four-letter word you'll ever hear" (Thaler and Koval 2006, 3–4). In this sense, being nice means moving forward with confidence in the notion that placing other people's needs and wants at the same level as yours will help achieve success for you and for them.

Similarly, William Baker and Michael O'Malley (2008) were among the first people to talk about kind leadership. Baker is the CEO of Educational Broadcasting Corp., and O'Malley is the acquiring editor for business, economics, and law at Yale University Press. They explain that kind leaders value and appreciate their employees, give honest feedback, encourage individual growth, communicate expectations, treat employees as volunteers, and act fairly and firmly. Kind leadership can therefore result in healthier, happier employees and positive organizational results in the long term. Empirical evidence backs up these claims and even suggests that kind leadership can improve employees' mental and physical health.

7

Swedish researchers at the Karolinska Institute set out to study the relationship between leadership style and ischemic heart disease

(IHD) among employees. They collected records of employee hospital admissions with a diagnosis of acute myocardial infarction or unstable angina, as well as deaths from IHD or cardiac arrest, over nine years. Leaders' positive behaviors, such as consideration for individual employees, supplying information and feedback, and promotion of employee participation and control, were rated by their subordinates (Nyberg et al. 2009). The results showed that higher leadership scores were associated with a lower incidence of heart disease. Kind leadership can be good for your heart!

Other research has shown that leadership behavior affects employee health mainly through stress. Kind behavior, perceived by followers as nonthreatening leadership, can significantly reduce stress levels. Brain-imaging studies show that when people perceive their social interactions with others as safe and secure, the threat-related activation in the amygdala is decreased, which in turn reduces their stress level (Norman et al. 2014). The opposite is also true. Unkind and excessively tough managers can put increased stress on their employees, which can have detrimental effects on health and productivity. For example, a study of 10,000 men and women working in the British civil service found that chronic exposure to work-related stress can significantly increase the risk of heart disease and type 2 diabetes. When employees work under a boss who creates unreasonable demands without providing enough latitude and control, immunity is decreased, and consumption of healthcare services goes through the roof (Chandola, Brunner, and Marmot 2006).

Management studies in healthcare and other fields tell a related story. Healthcare employees, directors, and executives believe that kindness is an important trait for effective, supportive leaders. For example, 38 percent of the respondents in my survey chose kindness (from a list of 20 traits) as a characteristic of the one leader they have observed to be the most successful, while 45 percent indicated that the leader who has had the most positive influence on their career was also kind. (See the appendix at the end of the book for the complete results.) In 2008, the American Management Association (AMA) conducted a survey of its members to examine how a boss's character affects employee performance and retention rates. About 75 percent of the respondents characterized their boss as kind, whereas 14 percent described their boss as a bully. When asked whether they plan to work for their company for a long time, 84 percent of the employees reporting to a kind boss said yes, but only 47 percent of those who reported to a bully agreed. Similarly, 70 percent of the employees who reported to a kind boss said that they worked as hard as they could, but only 54 percent of those who reported to a bully agreed that they did the same. These results clearly show how the relationship between employees and their leaders affects performance, productivity, and even bottom-line results. "It's the law of reciprocity: When a manager shows concern, his or her employees, in turn, support the manager. They do this by putting forth a maximum effort, being more dedicated to the organization, and by helping to achieve corporate goals," commented Edward Reilly, the then-president and CEO of AMA (AMA 2008).

Similarly, a recent study conducted in a long-term healthcare facility examined the culture of caring and kindness among employees. Authors Sigal Barsade and Olivia O'Neill coin the term *companionate love* to describe situations "when colleagues who are together day in and day out, ask and care about each other's work and even nonwork issues" (Maxwell 2016, 46). These employees are careful of each other's feelings and show compassion when things aren't going well. They demonstrate their caring through small acts such as bringing someone a cup of coffee or just listening if another needs to talk. The findings showed that this type of culture had a positive effect on employees' emotional and behavioral outcomes such as absenteeism, burnout, teamwork, and overall satisfaction. Interestingly, that culture of companionate love rippled out from staff to influence patients and their families. When employees treated each other with kindness, patients' quality of life, measured in terms of comfort, dignity, satisfaction with the food, and spiritual fulfillment, also improved significantly, and many of them had fewer trips to the emergency room (Barsade and O'Neill 2014).

The positive effects of kind leaders and cultures are therefore obvious in the workplace, but kindness on its own may not be enough. As discussed in chapter 3, the most effective leaders are those who are able to combine strength and determination with compassion and kindness. In a 2013 *Harvard Business Review* article, Amy Cuddy, Matthew Kohut, and John Neffinger argue that when employees evaluate their leaders, they look mainly at two characteristics: how lovable they are (i.e., their warmth, communion, trustworthiness) and how fearsome they are (i.e., their strength, competence). These traits are important because they answer two critical questions for people in relation to their leader: "What are this person's intentions toward me?" and "Is he or she capable of acting on those intentions?" (Cuddy, Kohut, and Neffinger 2013).

Psychological research shows that love and fear typically account for more than 90 percent of the variance in positive or negative impressions of others. Cuddy, Kohut, and Neffinger posit that leaders who project strength before establishing trust can cause fear among their followers, which typically leads to a number of dysfunctional behaviors. Fear is a "hot" emotion that can have long-lasting effects on employees, including reductions in cognitive potential, creativity, and problem-solving efforts, as well as disengagement. Because of this, they reason that "the way to influence—and to lead—is to begin with warmth" (Cuddy, Kohut, and Neffinger 2013). As warmth, trust, and communication are facilitated, ideas are absorbed and leaders can exercise more influence. A boss's nod, smile, or open gesture can signal to her followers that she is pleased with their company and attentive to their concerns. She shows them that she hears them, understands them, and can be trusted by them.

But warmth by itself isn't enough to lead. Leaders judged as warm—but incompetent or weak—tended to elicit pity and lack of respect. Therefore, the best way to gain influence is to combine warmth and strength, which can lead to admiration. When leaders feel a sense of personal strength, they can be more open, less threatened, and less threatening, especially under stress. This confidence and calm, in turn, can help to project warmth and authenticity to their followers.

Similar results were found by leadership development consultants Jack Zenger and Joseph Folkman in their study of 160,000 employees working for 30,000 leaders at hundreds of companies around the world. Zenger and Folkman identify two types of leaders: *drivers* and *enhancers*. They describe drivers as adept at establishing high standards, getting their employees to stretch for goals that they didn't think they could achieve, and keeping them focused on these goals. On the other hand, enhancers focus on staying in touch with the issues and concerns of employees, giving them honest but helpful feedback, developing them, and maintaining their trust (Zenger and Folkman 2013). Employees in the study were asked to rate themselves on engagement and commitment. Then they were asked to rate, on a scale of 1–5, to what degree they felt their leaders fit the profiles for enhancers and drivers. Only 8.9 percent of employees working for drivers and 6.7 percent of those working for enhancers rated themselves as highly engaged and committed. But 68 percent of the employees working for leaders they rated as both effective enhancers and strong drivers scored in the top on overall engagement (Zenger and Folkman 2013). The authors conclude that being tough but not nice, or the other way around, isn't enough to improve employee engagement. Leaders need to be both nice *and* tough.

8

What these studies point to is that different leaders can fall at different places on a continuum of traits, ranging from very kind and purely compassionate to extremely tough and determined. "Clearly, we were asking the wrong question when we set out to determine which approach was best. Leaders need to think in terms of 'and' not 'or'" (Zenger and Folkman 2013). Leaders who are considerate, trusting, and collaborative, but who also demand a great deal from their employees, can be highly effective in keeping them engaged.

Strong leaders who establish high standards shouldn't be afraid of the nice guy label. Kind leaders shouldn't think of challenging goals as incompatible with their leadership style. "The two approaches are like the oars of a boat. Both need to be used with equal force to maximize the engagement of direct reports," concluded Zenger and Folkman (2013).

Chade-Meng Tan (2010, 165), the Google engineer we met in chapter 3, makes a similar point when he suggests that "it is possible to understand another person at both an intellectual and visceral level with kindness and still respectfully disagree." According to him, we can make tough decisions while still being kind. He contends that some leaders convince themselves that when they have to make a decision that might hurt somebody's interest, they shouldn't bring kindness to the situation. They believe that kindness will only make the decision tougher. But Tan has found this belief to be untrue. Making tough decisions with no kindness may be the easy way out in the short term, but appearing cold and indifferent can create resentment and mistrust, which can have long-term negative effects. Instead, treating people with kindness and empathy in tough situations can help leaders better negotiate and manage concerns, which creates trust and understanding in the long run. Tan calls this approach "being tough without being an SOB" (Tan 2010, 165).

One of the hardest situations that a leader can find herself in is firing a subordinate. Most leaders develop close relationships over years of working with their team members, so having to terminate them can present significant heartache. Managers believe that these situations shouldn't be taken lightly—being fired is a significant life event for the person being let go. Bob Shaw agrees, but he has a unique approach to managing termination events. Bob is a former president of Norton Cancer Institute in Louisville, Kentucky. Prior to that, he held several high-level leadership positions, most notably at the MD Anderson Cancer Center. Over the course of his career, he has had to fire his fair share of executives and employees. Bob is a regular guest speaker in my Human Resources in Healthcare course. Every year, I invite him to talk to young graduate students about how to best handle terminations.

At the beginning of the class, Bob asks the students, "What is the most important factor to consider when terminating someone?" Answers typically focus on legal issues, safety, compensation, and so on. To their surprise, he says that, for him, the most important thing is to maintain the self-esteem and dignity of the person being terminated. He argues that even as a leader must share a decision that will deprive an employee of his main source of livelihood, she has to do it in a caring way. She must make sure that the individual being fired is offered the necessary support and resources to launch his career somewhere else.

But that doesn't mean going soft and apologizing. On the contrary, Bob keeps the conversation short and straight to the point. "I tell my HR [human resources] representative, if I am in there for longer than seven minutes, that means that I am in trouble, so please intervene to give me an exit opportunity," Bob explains (Shaw 2014). That, in a nutshell, represents Bob's leadership style: caring and kind but precise and strong. This style extends to his approach to dealing with his team. "I believe in the importance of caring for your team members. This relates to building leadership teams at the top, developing them, communicating with them. I call this 'unconditional love,' which is not typically talked about in business." Unconditional love applies even when firing someone—he may not be a good fit for your organization, but barring fraud, illegal acts, or unethical behavior, you still want to support him in his next career move to make sure he's successful in the long run (Shaw 2014).

9

Back to *Divergent*. The main character in the series is a young woman called Beatrice. Beatrice was born into the selfless Abnegation faction, but she always hated to show her weakness.

At the age of 16, her aptitude test shows that she is *divergent*, which means that she doesn't entirely fit into one faction and could choose a new one. To the surprise of her parents, Beatrice decides to join the Dauntless group, which she feels fits best with her personality. Under the new name Tris, she engages in exhilarating adventures that allow her to show her immense strength. But even in her new dog-eat-dog environment, she always remains kind inside, helping her fellow recruits when she can.

Let's reflect on some of the lessons that we've learned in this chapter. Kind leadership isn't the same as softness. To be kind, you have to be strong, confident, and competent. Also, kind leadership means being honest. It means providing candid feedback, both positive and negative. It means delivering a hard message, but in a humane way. As a healthcare leader, if your employees mess up, make mistakes, or take actions that might jeopardize patient care, kind leadership requires you to pull them aside and have a serious talk with them. Without using fear and intimidation, you help them see where they went wrong, and what the consequences of their actions are. If they keep repeating these actions, you have to be kind and strong enough to tell them that their job may not be the right fit for them.

Kind leadership is therefore not for the weak or lazy. It requires courage, time, and effort. You have to slow down and go out of your own way to lend a hand, say a word of encouragement, or listen. You have to be honest and to point out the problems. You have to take the time from your busy day to coach others and to mentor them toward success. And you have to be prepared to make tough and unpopular decisions.

REFERENCES

Aigner, G. 2011. *Leadership Beyond Good Intentions: What It Takes to Really Make a Difference.* Crows Nest, Australia: Allen & Unwin.

American Management Association (AMA). 2008. "American Management Association Survey Shows How the Boss's Character Affects Employee Productivity, Retention." *Corp!* Published October 20. www.corpmagazine.com/human-resources/the -peformance-premium-of-kindness/.

AZBio. 2017. "Dignity Health Survey Shows Humankindness Matters." Accessed March 13. www.azbio.org/dignity -humankindness.

Baker, W., and M. O'Malley. 2008. *Leading with Kindness: How Good People Consistently Get Superior Results.* New York: AMACOM.

Barsade, S. G., and O. A. O'Neill. 2014. "What's Love Got to Do with It? A Longitudinal Study of the Culture of Companionate Love and Employee and Client Outcomes in the Long-Term Care Setting." *Administrative Science Quarterly* 59 (4): 551–98.

Bohn, L. 2017. "Being Kind When It's Seen as a Weakness." *Tiny Buddha.* Accessed March 13. http://tinybuddha.com/blog /being-kind-when-its-seen-as-a-weakness/.

Brenoff, A. 2014. "What We Can Learn from the Man Who Runs The 'World's Happiest Company.'" *Huffington Post.* Published January 29. www.huffingtonpost.com/2014/01/29/worlds-best -company_n_4655292.html.

———. 2013. "8 Reasons Why Employees Never Want to Leave This Amazing Company." *Huffington Post.* November 18. www.huffingtonpost.com/2013/11/18/best-places-to -work_n_4240370.html.

Chandola, T., E. Brunner, and M. Marmot. 2006. "Chronic Stress at Work and the Metabolic Syndrome: Prospective Study." *British Medical Journal* 332 (7540): 521–25.

Crowley, M. 2013. "How SAS Became the World's Best Place to Work." *Fast Company.* Published January 22. www.fastcompany. com/3004953/how-sas-became-worlds-best-place-work.

Cuddy, A. J. C., M. Kohut, and J. Neffinger. 2013. "Connect, Then Lead." *Harvard Business Review*. Published July-August. https://hbr.org/2013/07/connect-then-lead.

Dignity Health. 2013. "We Should Never Cut, Ration, or Restrict Humanity." *Business on the Rise*. No date. www.hendersonchamber.com/os/resources/media/Rise_Insert_V04.pdf.

Edelman, R. C., T. R. Hiltabiddle, and C. C. Manz. 2008. *Nice Guys Can Get the Corner Office: Eight Strategies for Winning in Business Without Being a Jerk*. New York: Portfolio.

Greensweig, G. 2016. Personal interview. June 20.

———. 2014. "Why Practicing Medicine with Kindness Matters." *Becker's Hospital Review*. Published March 25. www.beckershospitalreview.com/hospital-management-administration/why-practicing-medicine-with-kindness-matters.html.

Hobbes, T. 2010. *Leviathan, or, The Matter, Forme, and Power of a Common-Wealth Ecclesiasticall and Civill*. New Haven, CT: Yale University Press.

Jazwiec, L. 2009. *Eat THAT Cookie! Make Workplace Positivity Pay Off . . . for Individuals, Teams, and Organizations*. Pensacola, FL: Fire Starter Publishing.

Maxwell, C. I. 2016. *Lead Like a Guide: How World-Class Mountain Guides Inspire Us to Be Better Leaders*. Westport, CT: Praeger.

Mitchell, J. 2008. *Hug Your People: The Proven Way to Hire, Inspire, and Recognize Your Employees and Achieve Remarkable Results*. New York: Hachette Books.

Norman, L., N. Lawrence, A. Iles, A. Benattayallah, and A. Karl. 2014. "Attachment-Security Priming Attenuates Amygdala Activation to Social and Linguistic Threat." *Social Cognitive and Affective Neuroscience* 10 (6): 832–39.

Nyberg, A., L. Alfredsson, T. Theorell, H. Westerlund, J. Vahtera, and M. Kivimäki. 2009. "Managerial Leadership and Ischaemic

Heart Disease Among Employees: The Swedish WOLF Study." *Occupational and Environmental Medicine* 66: 51–55.

Phillips, A., and B. Taylor. 2009. *On Kindness*. New York: Farrar, Straus, and Giroux.

Roth, V. 2017. "Faction Manifestos." Divergent Fans. Accessed March 27. http://divergentfans.net/page/faction-manifestos.

Seppälä, E. 2014. "The Hard Data on Being a Nice Boss." *Harvard Business Review*. Published November 24. https://hbr.org/2014/11/the-hard-data-on-being-a-nice-boss.

Shaw, B. 2014. Personal interview. November 11.

Tan, C. 2010. *Search Inside Yourself: The Unexpected Path to Achieving Success, Happiness (and World Peace)*. New York: HarperOne.

Tenney, M., and J. Gordon. 2014. *Serve to Be Great: Leadership Lessons from a Prison, a Monastery, and a Boardroom*. Hoboken, NJ: Wiley.

Thaler, L. K., and R. Koval 2006. *The Power of Nice: How to Conquer the World with Kindness*. New York: Crown Business.

Zenger, J., and J. Folkman. 2013. "Nice or Tough: Which Approach Engages Employees Most?" *Harvard Business Review*. Published September 11. https://hbr.org/2013/09/nice-or-tough-what-engages-emp.

CHAPTER 5

Generosity

1

HAMDI ULUKAYA WAS born in the small Turkish town of Ilic, which is located in the Kurdish region of Anatolia. Most of Ilic's 1,000 inhabitants are shepherds. Ulukaya's father, and his father before him, tended sheep and goats in the mountains and used their milk to make cheese and yogurt (Gross 2013). Ulukaya doesn't know his real birth date—only that he was born when his family was coming down with the herd from the mountains at the end of the summer, as opposed to going up at the beginning of the spring (Mead 2013).

In 1994, Ulukaya traveled to the United States to study English with only $3,000 in his pocket. Shortly after finishing school, he came across junk mail advertising the sale of an old yogurt factory in New Berlin, New York. The following day he toured the facility and decided to turn it into a strained yogurt (often called "Greek yogurt") factory, against his lawyer's best advice. With the help of a government loan, he reopened the facility in 2005 and brought a master yogurt maker from Turkey. He called his new company *Chobani*, the Turkish word for shepherd (Gross 2013). The rest, as they say, is history.

In five short years, Chobani became the leading yogurt brand in the United States, and Ulukaya one of the richest people on the planet. Contrary to common wisdom, Americans fell in love with Chobani's strained yogurt. "I've always loved yogurt—the thick kind I grew up eating in Turkey, where my mother made it from scratch on our family's dairy farm. When I moved to the United States . . . I found American yogurt to be disgusting—too sugary and watery," remarked Ulukaya a few years later (Ulukaya 2013).

But the secret behind his rapid success in building a billion-dollar company does not just lie in the yogurt itself. It goes much deeper, into the culture that he has created at his company. "From the beginning, I tried to treat everybody right," Ulukaya says. "We paid everyone well above minimum wage. Everybody in our plant gets the same holidays as everybody in the office. Our entire company—hourly or salaried—would get full health care, retirement plans" (Grenoble 2016). The culture that Ulukaya established at Chobani is built on generosity and kindness. Every Thanksgiving, each employee gets a free turkey and a bucket of feta cheese. In the summer of 2012, Ulukaya paid to take Chobani's founding five employees to watch the Olympic Games in London. When some staff once had to work a night shift on Christmas, he brought them prime rib for dinner and served it to them himself (Mead 2013).

Ulukaya's generosity extends beyond his employees. Realizing that New Berlin didn't have a functioning baseball field and that the Little League kids had to be driven around the area and play their games away, he invested $200,000 in a new high-quality ballpark that made the community proud. More significant, during the height of the refugee crisis in the Middle East in 2016, Chobani announced that it would start hiring refugees to help them resettle. Today, 30 percent of Chobani's workforce comprises refugees from 11 countries (Grenoble 2016). The company provides transportation to and from work and hires translators to help them better communicate with their coworkers. "The minute a refugee has a job, that's the minute they stop being a refugee," observes Ulukaya (Gelles 2016).

2

The idea of generosity in leadership can probably be credited to retired AT&T executive Robert Greenleaf, who introduced the concept of *servant leadership* in 1977. Greenleaf argues that servant leaders focus primarily on the growth and well-being of people and the communities to which they belong. While traditional leadership generally involves the accumulation and exercise of power by one person at the top of the pyramid, servant leadership is different. The servant leader shares power, puts the needs of others first, and helps people develop and perform to the highest degree possible. Greenleaf outlines ten characteristics of servant leadership. Of these, three are especially important for us in this chapter: empathy, healing, and commitment to the growth of people (Greenleaf 1977). Servant leaders strive to understand and empathize with followers. They assume good intentions and accept and recognize their followers for their special and unique spirit. In addition, they recognize that they have an opportunity to transform those with whom they come into contact. Servant leaders try to do everything in their power to nurture the growth of their followers. They make funds available for personal and professional development, take a personal interest in the ideas and suggestions of others, encourage involvement in decision making, and even actively assist laid-off employees in finding other positions (Greenleaf 1977).

Servant leadership was later picked up by famed author and management expert Ken Blanchard. He models his leadership approach after the example of Jesus Christ and advocates for a change in the heart of the leader that can help her shift from serving her own interests to serving others. Blanchard admits that the concept of servant leadership is often misunderstood. When he talks to managers about how they can become servant leaders, many of them are skeptical. They assume that under this model, employees get to decide what, when, where, and how—which does not sound like leadership for them. Rather, it "sounds more like the inmates are running the prison" (Blanchard 1995). Blanchard explains that there is a difference between the visionary part and the implementation part of leadership. Servant leaders still set the vision, as well as the direction the organization takes in order to achieve its goals. They decide on the ideal future and provide direction to get closer to that future. But once the direction is set, figuring out how it should be executed is up to the employees, with the support of their leaders. When it comes to implementation, servant leaders facilitate, nurture, and support, rather than set rigid rules and policies. That requires listening to employees, praising them, encouraging them, and helping them win.

Along the same lines, former Medtronic CEO Bill George advances the concept of authentic leadership. Among other qualities, George feels that authentic leaders genuinely desire to serve others through their leadership and are more interested in empowering the people they lead to make a difference than they are in power, money, or prestige. They're guided by their passion and compassion, as well as by their logical minds (George 2003).

3

Mark Crowley has decades of experience as a senior leader for regional and national financial institutions. He worked most of his career in a cutthroat environment characterized by hostility and heartlessness. Surprisingly, he developed a servant leadership approach that he describes in his influential book *Lead from the Heart*. Consider how Crowley talks about his style:

> What I chose to do is really basic and fundamental—but quite uncommon in business. As a hard-charging business leader, and as a man, I nurtured and supported the human needs in people so they could perform to their greatest potential. I did this all unconsciously at first and all my teams excelled. For many years, I took the success for

granted and didn't really connect the dots. But after several years had passed and I had the experience of leading myriad business units and teams of people, it became quite evident that the leadership practices I had implemented . . . were influencing people to be remarkably engaged and high achieving. (Crowley 2011, xii)

Crowley recognizes the challenges of raising these kinds of issues in the business world. Leading from the heart is typically thought of as being soft and sentimental—qualities diametrically opposed to cost-cutting and profit-maximization efforts. Yet, in his experience, his employees had achieved outstanding results because he recognized their potential, supported them, and helped them find meaning and fulfillment in their work. He has no doubt that it was indeed the heart-to-heart connections that he made with them that drove their achievements (Crowley 2011).

Why do leaders usually hesitate to make generous personal connections with their employees? The main barrier, Crowley argues, comes from traditional leadership theory, which suggests that management must not be concerned with the personal issues affecting workers. Because of this limited view, leaders fear that by connecting more personally with employees, they might complicate the leader–worker relationship. This connection, in turn, might lead to loss of control, compromised ability to implement change, and reduced productivity. Crowley recognizes that while it is inappropriate for leaders to fraternize with subordinates and to become too involved in their private lives, many leaders have taken this idea of keeping their distance from employees to the extreme (Crowley 2011).

One important aspect that differentiates generous leaders is that they have an *abundance mentality*. They believe that the universe has no limits on the number of people who can be successful, and that everyone, not just a few, can achieve, grow, and thrive. They also maintain that if they give of themselves—their time, knowledge, and help—others will inevitably give more. On the other hand, individuals with a *scarcity mentality* have a belief that we live in a world where everything is limited. They reason that because opportunity is limited, competition is the only way to go forward. If they teach others and share their knowledge, they worry that they'll inherently diminish themselves and become less powerful. If they help others to grow, develop, and progress, that will lead others to catapult over them in recognition, compensation, and career opportunities (Crowley 2011).

4

If you're still feeling a bit skeptical about the idea of servant leadership, you're not alone. When the Cleveland Clinic decided in 2008 to revamp its organizational culture based on the principle, many of its executives were unconvinced. For example, the chief operating officer at the time insisted that servant leadership "will never work here" and specifically told the other executives leading the effort, "I'm not going to let you take 40,000 people down this path" (Patmchak 2015, 41). But the story of the Cleveland Clinic offers solid evidence that servant leadership actually works.

It's common knowledge that the Cleveland Clinic is one of the best organizations in the world, if not the best, at delivering high-quality clinical care, especially for cardiac patients. However, in 2008, its leaders started to realize that despite its reputation for excellence, the clinic's patient experience was not on par with its clinical outcomes. According to Dr. Toby Cosgrove, the outspoken CEO of the organization, "Patients were coming to us for the clinical excellence, but they did not like us very much" (Patmchak 2015, 37). The scores earned by the clinic on the HCAHPS (Hospital Consumer Assessment of Healthcare Providers and Systems) survey showed as much. Another area in which the clinic was struggling was employee satisfaction and engagement, as many people felt unappreciated and undervalued. The organization received mediocre scores on the Gallup employee engagement survey, especially on four survey statements in particular: (1) "In the last seven days,

I have received recognition or praise for doing good work;" (2) "At work my opinions seem to count;" (3) "There is someone at work who encourages my development;" and (4) "I have a best friend at work" (Patmchak 2015, 45).

To address both patient satisfaction and employee engagement, the clinic's leaders decided that a radical culture change was necessary. They put together a plan based on the principles of servant leadership. The changes started with a soft launch during which the concept was gradually introduced to key members of the executive leadership team in small group presentations. While many were excited, the strategies were not universally accepted. Physicians, especially, struggled with the new way of thinking. One surgeon said, "Hey, in my OR [operating room], I'm in charge. Period. That's the way it has to be, and that's the way it is. And now you expect me to also be a servant leader? Come on" (Patmchak 2015, 41). Despite the resistance, the principles managed to trickle down to all levels of the organization. This phase was followed by servant leadership training and coaching for all 65 clinical and nonclinical executives and to more than 400 directors throughout the clinic.

Since 2009, a large number of initiatives have been put in place to make sure that the leaders have the necessary tools and that the servant leadership principles are embedded throughout the culture of the organization. For example, servant leadership competencies were specified and integrated in the periodic leadership development programs. Champions were selected throughout the organization to receive extensive training and ensure implementation in their departments and units. Servant leadership metrics were used to evaluate the performance of leaders, and executive rounding was initiated to recognize caregivers and listen to employee and patient concerns (Patmchak 2015). How did these changes affect the outcomes? HCAHPS scores that were lingering in the fortieth percentile in 2008 jumped to the eightieth percentile in 2013. Employee engagement rates also jumped from 43 percent to 87 percent over the same period, with significant increases in the four areas highlighted earlier. In 2008, for every disengaged employee, 2.57 were engaged, and by 2013, there were 10.2—well above the world-class ratio of 1:9.57 (Patmchak 2015). Dr. Cosgrove could relax knowing that, through servant leadership principles, patient satisfaction and engagement scores were starting to catch up with the clinical metrics.

5

Let's examine the idea of the generous leader more in depth. In chapter 3, we talked about compassion in leadership. What makes generosity different from compassion is that generosity is compassion in action. It requires leaders to go beyond care and empathy and to engage in specific behaviors. Generous leaders give their time, energy, talents, and money. All leaders are typically preoccupied with strategies and big-picture ideas, which is what they get paid to do. But being generous also requires focusing on the people around them and taking the time to connect genuinely. In doing so, generous leaders share their wisdom, knowledge, and experience—they spread what they know with the goal of helping others improve (Bonner 2014).

Time is always a rare commodity, especially at the highest level. Leaders are typically very protective of their time, giving access to only a handful of privileged people. But generous leaders slow down so they can be unhurried and mindful in their daily interactions with others. They make intentional eye contact, and when they ask, for example, about how someone's family is doing, they actually listen to the answer. They show others that they consider them important, and they choose words and actions that communicate that they consider employees' work and lives significant (Daskal 2015).

Moreover, they stand up for their people, and they show that they're on their workers' side with support and assistance. They stay late to help others with a project approaching its deadline. If an individual merits a chance, or a second chance, or is deserving but not well positioned to be noticed, generous leaders open doors, create the right circumstances, and help that person achieve his goals. They seek out those who have a need and take actions to address that need (Kotrla 2014). For example, if you're an early careerist, a generous leader will bring you to high-level meetings you wouldn't otherwise be involved in or take you to a working lunch at which new projects are being discussed.

When treated in a negative way, generous leaders act forcefully but also have the ability to forgive without holding long-term grudges. When individuals or groups succeed, generous leaders lavish them with acknowledgments, celebrating achievements publicly while also expressing appreciation in private. They give the credit away because they understand the value of creating a sense of shared success. Just as important, they also look for opportunities to reward high performers financially. Jack Welch, the celebrated former CEO of General Electric, believes that effective leaders have a "generosity gene" and want to see their employees do well and grow within the company. He argues that these leaders love to give praise and enjoy seeing their people grow. "When they give a raise, they're turned on; when [their employees are] given stock options or stock, they can't be more excited," he observes (Welch 2015).

In a recent article, Welch elaborates on this idea by reflecting on how leader generosity can affect employee engagement:

> Employee engagement . . . is something that is in the hands of every leader, every day—whether you're managing one, ten, a thousand, or ten thousand. [Leaders should] ask themselves these questions: Has my team really bought into the mission? Do they understand where we're going, and why we're doing what we do to get there? Equally important, or perhaps more important, have I made it clear to them what's in it for them when we get there? Am I celebrating their achievements, reaching the milestones we've established? Am I coaching them in a constructive manner so that they feel I have their back? Do they always

know where they stand? Have I given them the freedom and the authority to raise these same questions with their team? (Welch 2016)

Welch isn't a soft leader by any stretch of the imagination. In fact, most people who have worked with him were overwhelmed by his intensity and strong personality. When confronting a problem that annoyed him, "he [came] on like a battery of howitzers, flattening all opposition." He walked into meetings warning, "We've got a disaster here" before even saying hello (Tichy and Sherman 2001, 17). He looked people straight in the eye and told them exactly why he thought they were wrong. But if they stood up for themselves and talked back, he listened to them. If they could solve problems and achieve results, he supported them forever.

John Paul DeJoria is a generous successful leader of a different kind. DeJoria created not one, but two billion-dollar companies: Paul Mitchell Systems and Patron Tequila. On the CNBC show *Follow the Leader*, business journalist Farnoosh Torabi followed him around for a few days and was surprised to find him very positive, even in the face of challenges. His team meetings were amazingly upbeat and stress-free. Wearing a ponytail and an all-black outfit, and working from his home office in Los Angeles, the 71-year-old is the picture of the relaxed CEO. When Torabi asked him what type of boss he is, he articulated a profound philosophy: "I am not a boss, we're socialist, we all work together. We have been around for 36 years and my turnover is less than a hundred people. I've worked for people in the past who were 'bosses' and they weren't nice at all. 'Do this because I said so.' I made sure that I treated my people the way I wished these people had treated me at the time. The more I make, the more I get to give back. Success unshared is failure" (Torabi 2016). While Welch and DeJoria may have drastically different leadership approaches, what they have in common is that they understand the importance of investing in their people and developing them.

Stan Hupfeld is probably the only healthcare executive in America with the distinction of having a charter school named after him. Stan is the retired CEO of INTEGRIS Health System, one of the largest hospital systems in Oklahoma, and many consider him the embodiment of the generous leader in healthcare. He has held several executive positions over a long and successful work history that saw him earn several awards and accolades for himself and his organizations. Throughout his career, he focused on giving opportunities for advancement to people in his organizations, especially those from minority groups and impoverished backgrounds. Since his retirement in 2010, he has continued his generosity by serving as executive-in-residence at the graduate program in healthcare administration at Trinity University. In this role, he spends time with students, sharing his vast knowledge, advising and coaching, and providing feedback on presentations and interviews.

Corinne Smith, a former leader in several healthcare organizations and now a partner in a healthcare law firm, started her career working for Stan as an administrative resident at INTEGRIS. "Stan spoiled me for the rest of my career," she observes. "As the CEO, he was so down-to-earth. He knew the names of everyone, he shook hands with janitors, he was so kind, honest, almost like a father figure," she says nostalgically. As the resident, Stan allowed Corinne to accompany him to all the meetings that he attended. "I followed him everywhere and saw how he dealt with others. He listened to everyone, he had an ego but he kept it from people, he took counsel from others. I haven't worked with anyone like him" (Smith 2016).

While he was at the Trinity campus a short while ago, I sat down to talk to Stan and asked him about generosity in leadership. His eyes lit up as he explained, "In leadership, there is an element of being seen. But it is easy to get wrapped up in urgent problems and forget about the important ones. As leaders, it is easy to trick ourselves that we are busy with meetings, phone calls, and budgets, but the most important things are the morale of your employees, your mission, keeping your word" (Hupfeld 2014). I asked him how busy CEOs can find the time to be generous. He leaned forward in his chair and clarified, "By counseling an employee with a problem, talking to them, developing them. People admire personal generosity. The admirable qualities that people like in leaders and will follow them for are generosity, truthfulness, and humility, especially when things are difficult. You have to *love* your employees" (Hupfeld 2014).

If you're starting to imagine Stan as a teddy bear, you're a bit off. He was a member of the 1963 National Championship football team from the University of Texas, Austin. Many people would describe him as "tough as nails," especially physicians who have sat across the table from him. Corinne describes how Stan dealt with them: "In negotiations he was very calm. I never once heard him yell at someone. When dealing with aggressive doctors, he would get all the facts before talking to them; he never tried to manipulate them. He disarmed them by being calm and steady. But if they asked for something that was unrealistic, he just told them that he couldn't do it" (Smith 2016). Stan admits that he was especially tough on doctors, even the difficult ones, but at the same time he admired them for achieving their medical training, "something few of us are smart enough or tough enough to achieve" (Hupfeld 2016).

To hear Stan talk about love in the workplace was surprising to me. But as you may have noticed by now, leaders are becoming more comfortable talking about love in business these days. A few years ago, a book by the name *Love Is the Killer App* came on the management scene. In it, Tim Sanders, a former Yahoo executive, encourages people to share their intangibles (e.g., their knowledge, network, compassion). Those who are able to do that, he argues, can become a *lovecat*, a nice, smart person who succeeds in business and in life. Sanders explains that a lovecat becomes a rich source of information to all around him, is seen as a person with valuable insight, and is perceived as generous to a fault. Moreover, he's able to double his business intelligence in one year, triple his network of personal relationships in two years, and quadruple the number of colleagues in his life who love him like family. In short, the love-cat becomes "one of those amazing, outstanding people to whom everyone turns, who leads rather than follows, who never runs out of ideas, contacts, or friendship" (Sanders 2017).

Who doesn't want to become that guy? The driving force behind all of that, according to Sanders, is love. Love in the workplace, as unusual a concept as it may sound, can help companies grow and thrive. It can help leaders establish a sense of meaning and satisfaction in their work, which can help propel their careers.

7

I hope that by now you're expecting what will come next. Where is the evidence? The concepts of generosity and giving in the workplace and in life have received a lot of attention lately, especially with the publication of the remarkable book *Give and Take* by Adam Grant. Grant is a professor of organizational psychology at the Wharton School of Business at the University of Pennsylvania. He argues that there are three kinds of people in business: *givers*, *takers*, and *matchers*. Givers prefer to give more than they get, focus and act on the interest of others, and help others without expecting anything in return. Takers put their own interests ahead of others and believe the world is a competitive, brutal place. Matchers strive to preserve an equal balance of giving and getting and have relationships governed by an even exchange of favors. By drawing on research conducted in different industries, Grant set out to examine the evidence about who tends to do better at work—givers, takers, or matchers? (Grant 2014).

In a separate study of professional engineers in California, the participants rated one another on help received and given and then were evaluated on objective measures of performance. The worst-performing engineers were those who gave more than they received. Because they spent a lot of time helping others, these givers had the worst scores on the number of tasks, technical reports, and drawings they completed, in addition to making many errors, missing deadlines, and wasting money. However, and make sure you read this carefully: The best-performing engineers were *also* those who gave more than they received! So givers comprise the worst and best performers, while the takers and the matchers tended to be middle performers (Flynn 2003). The same pattern was observed in a study of 600 medical students in Belgium. The students who agreed with statements such as "I love to help others" and "I anticipate the needs of others" had the lowest exam grades. These givers allocated valuable time to helping their fellow students, sharing what they knew instead of studying more, which gave others a chance to outperform them on exams. But once again, the students with the highest grades were givers who agreed with these same statements (Lievens, Ones, and Dilchert 2009). The same conclusion was reached in a study involving salespeople in North Carolina, as well as studies across several other occupations: Givers land at the bottom and the top of the performance curve, while takers and matchers occupy the middle (Grant 2014). What's really going on?

Grant explains that there are two types of givers: those who give without any self-interest and end up burnt out, and those who give but are also self-interested, and end up achieving huge successes. The givers who end up losing (let's call them *pushovers*) tend to be nice in an extremely naive way: They give to others but forget about themselves. The givers who win (the *successful givers*) do better than others when they give while also being ambitious and focused on their own individual achievements. But unlike the takers, they achieve success without hurting others or stirring jealousy and vengefulness. In fact, when successful givers achieve important results, everyone else is rooting for them and supporting them—everyone else has, in one way or another, benefited from their generosity and good deeds. Grant makes the case that it's easier to win when you don't have a lot of enemies and everyone wants you to succeed (Grant 2014).

Consider this question: How can leaders be givers and still make hard decisions? Grant argues that making tough and sometimes unpopular decisions can be hard for givers who are always agreeable and polite. But leaders need to distinguish between being liked and being respected. Insufferable people pleasers never make the right decision because they constantly worry about being loved by everyone. Being respected means making decisions that are in the best interest of the organization.

8

Not only can giving be important in advancing your career, it can also benefit your health.

As we discussed in chapter 4, the negative effects of stress on health conditions and mortality are well documented in the scientific literature. To understand the relationship between giving, stress, and death, psychology researcher Michael Poulin and his colleagues studied a sample of older adults in Detroit, Michigan. First, they asked those individuals if they had experienced a stressful event in the past 12 months, such as serious non-life-threatening illness, burglary, job loss, financial difficulty, or death of a family member. They also asked the participants whether they had engaged in any unpaid activity directed toward helping friends, neighbors, or relatives who didn't live with them. These activities included transportation, errands, or shopping; housework; child care; and other tasks. The participants were asked to estimate the amount of time in hours they spent in those helping activities. Over a period of five years, the researchers tracked the participants' mortality and time to death by checking newspaper obituaries and monthly death records (Poulin et al. 2013).

Not surprisingly, stressful events were related to a 30 percent increase in mortality. But that applied only to individuals who didn't help others—such people demonstrated a direct relationship between suffering a serious setback and dying. However, for those who consistently gave rides to neighbors, ran errands for friends, or helped relatives with grocery shopping, stress didn't have any effect on mortality. Helping others has a buffering effect between stressful life events and death (Poulin et al. 2013). Being generous with time and effort, as it turns out, can actually save your life.

Let's dig below the surface and see how that works at the physiological level. Researchers Rachel Piferi and Kathleen Lawler investigated the relationship between giving and blood pressure. They measured blood pressure and heart rate for a group of study participants over a 24-hour period. They noticed that people who gave more social support to others had lower blood pressure and healthier hearts. Those same individuals also received more social support and had greater self-efficacy, higher self-esteem, less depression, and lower stress levels than people who gave less (Piferi and Lawler 2006). Other research using brain-imaging technology has shown that when people give money to charity, especially on a voluntary basis, the same pleasure-related centers in their brains light up as when they actually receive money. People can experience as much pleasure in giving as in receiving (Harbaugh, Mayr, and Burghart 2007). Leaders face considerable demands and stress in their jobs. Because giving can be so good for overall wellness, blood pressure, and heart health, current and future leaders should consider adopting generosity as a practice in their relationships with followers.

9

In this section we'll shift gears and comb through the evidence that relates leaders' generosity to individual and organizational performance. A study of managers in India examined whether leaders who were more self-sacrificing and altruistic were better at convincing followers to accept and internalize their vision. The results showed that leaders who were perceived as giving up or postponing personal interests and putting others' goals over their own were judged by others to be better transformational leaders—that is, leaders who created trust and inspired them to achieve long-term goals. This dynamic, in turn, helped improve followers' performance (Singh and Krishnan 2008).

Similarly, a study of Spanish firms examined leaders who put the interests of other people above their own, who did all they could to help people, who sacrificed their own interests to meet the needs of others, and who went beyond the call of duty to help. Those altruistic leaders were able to drive better customer retention, sales growth, profitability, and return on investment in their organizations than nonaltruistic leaders (Mallén et al. 2013).

Research by leadership coach Dennis Romig echoes these results. Romig has shown that the practices of servant leadership can help improve employee performance in organizations by 15–20 percent and work group productivity by 20–50 percent (Romig 2001). Similarly, a study of 1,500 firms from various industries showed that participative leadership practices enhance employee retention, increase productivity, and improve financial performance. In fact, each standard deviation in participative practices resulted in a $35,000–$78,000 spike in the company's market value per employee (Blanchard 2010). Being a generous leader is associated with improved organizational performance partly because it affects how a leader is perceived by those she works with. The way leaders come across to their employees is key to the type of relationship that they have and to the long-term success of the organization. Employees' perceptions of you as altruistic, selfish, approachable, or intimidating can have a serious impact on how they act in your presence as well as when you're not around.

The relationship between altruistic leader behavior and dominance and prestige in an organization is mixed. In an older study, researchers Charlie Hardy and Mark Van Vugt (2006) from the University of Kent in England tested several altruism hypotheses. They handed a group of college students a specific sum of money and gave them the choice of contributing some or all of that money to a private fund or a public fund under different scenarios. The students were then asked to rank each other on perceived status and influence and to choose an individual whom they deemed the most appropriate to be the group leader. Overall, altruistic individuals were granted more status by others than selfish ones: They were held in higher esteem, more respected, and more likely to be chosen as group leaders by teammates (Hardy and Van Vugt 2006).

However, more recent research on the issue shows different results. Investigators from Stanford University and Northwestern University have concluded that altruism can block leadership. How can that be? The setting was similar to the Hardy and Van Vugt study. Participants were divided into groups and provided game chips worth a specific sum of money. They were given the freedom to keep the chips to themselves, give them to their own group, or give them to another group. After different scenarios, the participants were asked to rate each other on dominance and prestige. Dominance relates to the use of intimidation, coercion, and fear to attain a social status, whereas prestige is based on altruistic achievements or having a sound character. They were also asked what type of person they would choose as a leader for tasks that could be achieved in the same group as well as those that required competing with another group. People with more prestige were chosen to lead internal tasks, whereas dominant individuals were chosen for tasks for which the groups had to compete. The most surprising finding, however, was that generous individuals who contributed to the benefit of both their group and other groups were rated lowest on both dominance and prestige (Nir et al. 2012).

Coauthor Robert Livingston, assistant professor of management and organizations at the Kellogg School of Management at Northwestern, comments,

> Do nice guys finish last? In competitive contexts, the answer is often yes. The reason that they finish last is because being nice, contributing costly resources to the group, acts of generosity—these all increase your prestige. Other people admire you and say, "Oh, that's really great. This is a kind person who's doing all these wonderful things."

But it decreases your dominance. It makes you look not so tough. Altruism is a double-edged sword. On the one hand, generous individuals are admired for their kindness, compassion, and willingness to help. On the other hand, they may be perceived as feeble "bleeding hearts" who lack the guts to make tough decisions that might advance the goals of the organization. (Kellogg Insight 2011)

So how do we make sense of this? As I've argued throughout this book, leadership is never an either-or situation: You have to be generous *and* strong. Leaders who are too soft, no matter how competent they are, may not be respected by others. But those who are too dominant and use only force to stay in power will likely be resented by their subordinates. As the evidence highlighted earlier suggests, both prestige and dominance are necessary for success in leadership.

10

Back to Hamdi Ulukaya. Ulukaya never relied on venture capitalists or private equity for his start-up business and has remained the sole owner of Chobani (Ulukaya 2013). In April of 2016, he made the extraordinary announcement that he was giving his employees awards worth up to 10 percent of the company, should it go public or be sold. Given the company's current valuation, these awards could be equivalent to $150,000–$1 million per employee, depending on seniority. In a memo, Ulukaya told his people that the award was not a gift but "a mutual promise to work together with a shared purpose and responsibility. How we built this company matters to me, but how we grow it matters even more. I want you to be a part of this growth—I want you to be the driving force of it" (McGregor 2016). When they received their white packets containing their awards, euphoric employees hugged and kissed the Turkish immigrant. Rich Lake, lead project manager and one of the original group of five employees hired by Ulukaya, remarked, "It's better than a bonus or a raise. It's the best thing because you're getting a piece of this thing you helped build" (Strom 2016).

In this chapter we've uncovered the importance of generosity among leaders such as Hamdi Ulukaya. Servant leadership, leading from the heart, and loving your employees imply that you care about your followers and that you go out of your way to appreciate and support them. This approach can pay dividends for your own health and career success and for your organization's success. Despite the overwhelming evidence, many people still hesitate to be generous in the workplace for fear of appearing weak or soft. In my survey of healthcare employees, managers, and executives, generosity was only the ninth-ranked trait of successful leaders (chosen by 29 percent) and the eighth-ranked trait of leaders who positively influenced their subordinates' careers (chosen by 35 percent). (See the appendix at the end of the book for the full results.)

Now is the time for healthcare leaders to acknowledge the importance of generosity. They need to realize that they're in a special position to give to others and to benefit the organization. Although they have limited time, numerous stakeholders to satisfy, and many requests to meet, they have two advantages that allow them to give more than others. First, it's easier for them "to multiply themselves and create networks of givers," as Adam Grant suggests (Buchanan 2013). They have the opportunity to build cultures in which giving is the norm and, as a result, to spread the giving to people around and below them. For example, leaders who act as mentors often encourage their mentees to develop people below them and start paying it forward. Second, it's a lot easier for leaders to attend short meetings with bursts of attention and energy that can have a lasting impact on others. Many people remember their first job when the big boss stopped by their desk, shook their hand, and asked questions that showed interest in them and their success. It probably lasted only three minutes, but it meant the world to them. As you climb the corporate ladder, remember that you can use your stature during short interactions to notice and recognize your employees. They'll always remember that, and they'll never let you down.

REFERENCES

Blanchard, K. 2010. *Leading at a Higher Level*. Upper Saddle River, NJ: Pearson Prentice Hall.

———. 1995. "One Minute Manager." *Quality Digest*. Published October. www.qualitydigest.com/oct/blanchrd.html.

Bonner, B. 2014. *Inspiring Generosity*. Boston: Wisdom Publications.

Buchanan, L. 2013. "Why the Most Successful Leaders Are Givers." *Inc.* Published April 5. www.inc.com/leigh-buchanan/adam-grant-leadership-give-and-take.html.

Crowley, M. 2011. *Lead from the Heart: Transformational Leadership for the 21st Century*. Bloomington, IN: Balboa Press.

Daskal, L. 2015. "10 Habits to Help You Become a More Generous Leader." *Inc.* Published August 31. www.inc.com/lolly-daskal/10-habits-on-how-to-become-a-more-generous-leader.html.

Flynn, F. 2003. "How Much Should I Give and How Often? The Effects of Generosity and Frequency of Favor Exchange on Social Status and Productivity." *Academy of Management Journal* 46 (5): 539–53.

Gelles, D. 2016. "For Helping Immigrants, Chobani's Founder Draws Threats." *New York Times*. Published October 31. www.nytimes.com/2016/11/01/business/for-helping-immigrants-chobanis-founder-draws-threats.html.

George, B. 2003. *Authentic Leadership: Rediscovering the Secrets to Creating Lasting Value*. San Francisco: Jossey-Bass.

Grant, A. 2014. *Give and Take: Why Helping Others Drives Our Success*. London: Penguin Books.

Greenleaf, R. 1977. *Servant Leadership: A Journey into the Nature of Legitimate Power and Greatness*. New York: Paulist Press.

Grenoble, R. 2016. "Chobani Hires Refugees and Treats Them Well. That Makes a Lot of People Angry." *Huffington*

Post. Published November 1. www.huffingtonpost.com/entry /chobani-ceo-refugee-immigrant-hamdi-ulukaya_us_58189 ac4e4b0990edc336cab.

Gross, D. 2013. "It's All Greek to Him: Chobani's Unlikely Success Story." *Newsweek.* Published June 12. www.newsweek .com/2013/06/12/its-all-greek-him-chobanis-unlikely-success -story-237526.html.

Harbaugh, W., U. Mayr, and D. Burghart. 2007. "Neural Responses to Taxation and Voluntary Giving Reveal Motives for Charitable Donations." *Science* 316 (5831): 1622–25.

Hardy, C., and M. Van Vugt. 2006. "Nice Guys Finish First: The Competitive Altruism Hypothesis." *Personality and Social Psychological Bulletin* 32 (10): 1402–13.

Hupfeld, S. 2016. E-mail correspondence with the author. December 21.

———. 2014. Personal interview. October 29.

Kellogg Insight. 2011. "Nice Guys Finish Last: Altruism May Be Rewarded with Prestige, But Seldom with Leadership." Published October 31. http://insight.kellogg.northwestern.edu /article/nice_guys_finish_last.

Kotrla, D. 2014. "13 Characteristics of a Generous Leader." Vanderbloemen Search Group. Published May 12. www.vanderbloemen .com/blog/13-characteristics-of-a-generous-leader.

Lievens, F., D. Ones, and S. Dilchert. 2009. "Personality Scale Validities Increase Throughout Medical School." *Journal of Applied Psychology* 94 (6): 1514–35.

Mallén, F., R. Chiva, J. Alegre, and J. Guinot. 2013. "Altruistic Leadership and Performance: The Mediating Role of Organizational Learning Capability." George Washington Graduate School of Education and Human Development. Published April. www .olkc2013.com.

McGregor, J. 2016. "How Chobani CEO Ensures That Employees Will Share in the Company's Success." *Los Angeles Times.* Published May 1. www.latimes.com/business/la-fi-on-leadership-chobani-20160430-story.html.

Mead, R. 2013. "Just Add Sugar: How an Immigrant from Turkey Turned Greek Yogurt into an American Snack Food." *New Yorker.* Published November 4. www.newyorker.com/magazine/2013/11/04/just-add-sugar.

Nir, H., E. Chou, T. Cohen, and R. Livingston. 2012. "Status Conferral in Intergroup Social Dilemmas: Behavioral Antecedents and Consequences of Prestige and Dominance." *Journal of Personality and Social Psychology* 102 (2): 351–66.

Patmchak, J. M. 2015. "Implementing Servant Leadership at Cleveland Clinic: A Case Study in Organizational Change." *Servant Leadership: Theory and Practice* 2 (1): 36–48.

Piferi, R., and K. Lawler. 2006. "Social Support and Ambulatory Blood Pressure: An Examination of Both Receiving and Giving." *International Journal of Psychophysiology* 62 (2): 328–36.

Poulin, M., S. Brown, A. Dillard, and D. Smith. 2013. "Giving to Others and the Association Between Stress and Mortality." *American Journal of Public Health* 103 (9): 1649–55.

Romig, D. 2001. *Side by Side Leadership.* Marietta, GA: Bard Press.

Sanders, T. 2017. "Love Is the Killer App." Accessed April 3. http://timsanders.com/love-is-the-killer-app/.

———. 2002. *Love Is the Killer App: How to Win Business and Influence Friends.* New York: Crown Business.

Singh, N., and V. Krishnan. 2008. "Self-sacrifice and Transformational Leadership: Mediating Role of Altruism." *Leadership and Organization Development Journal* 29 (3): 261–74.

Smith, C. 2016. Phone interview. August 29.

Strom, S. 2016. "At Chobani, Now It's Not Just the Yogurt That's Rich." *New York Times*. Published April 26. www.nytimes.com/2016/04/27/business/a-windfall-for-chobani-employees-stakes-in-the-company.html.

Tichy, N., and S. Sherman. 2001. *Control Your Destiny or Someone Else Will*. New York: Harper Business.

Torabi, F. 2016. "Five Habits of Billionaire John Paul DeJoria." CNBC. Published April 5. www.cnbc.com/2016/04/04/five-habits-of-billionaire-john-paul-dejoria.html.

Ulukaya, H. 2013. "Chobani's Founder on Growing a Start-Up Without Outside Investors." *Harvard Business Review*. Published October. https://hbr.org/2013/10/chobanis-founder-on-growing-a-start-up-without-outside-investors.

Welch, J. 2016. "The Number One New Year's Resolution Every Leader Should Make." LinkedIn. Published January 4. www.linkedin.com/pulse/number-one-new-years-resolution-every-leader-should-make-jack-welch.

———. 2015. "Jack and Suzy Welch on Generous Leadership." Yale School of Management. Published April 16. http://som.yale.edu/news/2015/04/jack-and-suzy-welch-generous-leadership.

PART 3

Applications

CHAPTER 6

Men and Women

Warning: The contents of this chapter are relevant to both men and women. Do not skip!

1

"In 1976 the Girl Scouts of America, one of our country's greatest institutions, was near collapse," began President Bill Clinton. He continued,

> Frances Hesselbein, a former volunteer from Johnstown, Pennsylvania, led them back, both in numbers and in spirit. She achieved not only the greatest diversity in the group's long history but also its greatest cohesion and, in so doing, became a model for us all. In her current role as the president of the Drucker Foundation for Nonprofit Management, she has shared her remarkable recipe for inclusion and excellence with countless organizations whose bottom line is measured not in dollars but in changed lives. Since Mrs. Hesselbein forbids the use of hierarchical words like "up" and "down" when she's around, I will call this pioneer for women, voluntarism, diversity, and opportunity not up but forward to be recognized. (Hesselbein 2011, ix)

The audience erupted in applause as President Bill Clinton introduced Frances Hesselbein at the White House East Room. On that day of January 15, 1998, Hesselbein was awarded the Presidential Medal of Freedom, the country's highest civilian award. Standing among other notable honorees, the woman felt humbled and overwhelmed. As she walked to the stage, she thought of her family and her childhood experiences. How did she go from a shy little girl in a small town to one of the most influential female leaders in the country?

Thirty years earlier, Hesselbein was a volunteer with the Talus Rock Girl Scout Council in Pennsylvania. One day, some members of the local council took her to lunch and tried to persuade her to take on the position of executive director of the council. After much convincing, she reluctantly accepted, but only "for six months while we look for a real leader" (Hesselbein 2011, 1). She ended up staying for six years. A few years later, she became the CEO of Girl Scouts of America. At the time, the organization was going through a very difficult period. Several challenges threatened its very existence: declining membership, decreased relevance, financial difficulties, and takeover plans from the Boy Scouts of America. Hesselbein faced these challenges without thinking of her role as the manager on top of a hierarchy. Rather, she presented herself as a leader who connected people in pursuit of a common mission. She banned the old hierarchy and involved as many heads and hands as possible. She took people out of their boxes and moved them into a more circular and fluid style of management that released their energy and spirit. She rededicated the organization to its long-term mission, which is to enable girls to reach their highest potential.

Hesselbein set forth a policy that everything the organization did could be challenged and changed, as long as it met three basic tests. First, any new activity should fit squarely with the mission. Second, the organization should have the resources to do that activity better than anyone else. Third, the activity should make sense financially for the organization. As Peter Drucker, the "father of management" and her longtime friend, often said, the foundation for doing good is doing well. Under her leadership, the organization drastically increased its membership and volunteer workforce, tripled its racial and ethnic diversity ratios, and resumed its crucial educational and developmental role for girls of all backgrounds (Hesselbein 2011).

Hesselbein's leadership style, which focused on people as the greatest organizational asset, was a breath of fresh air in the Girl Scouts. For her, "leadership is a matter of how to be, not how to do it" (Hesselbein 2002, 32). To lead isn't just to know all the how-tos or to have the skills and master the practices. Rather, leadership is about character, mind-set, values, and principles. She argues that cutting-edge practical knowledge changes with times and markets, but character remains the same. An important aspect of character for Hesselbein is good manners. "Tough leaders . . . who saved their manners for their social lives and believed in barking orders and the power of command and control, are now part of history," she writes (Hesselbein 2002, 33). In their place are leaders who show, through their words and actions, their appreciation and respect for people who work with them. She maintains that effective leaders know that good manners are critical to developing strong workplace relationships, building effective teams, managing a diverse workforce, and dealing with customer needs. These good manners don't come from patterned niceness, but rather from a leader's genuine appreciation of the people she works with.

While some might dismiss this as soft management, Hesselbein challenged anyone to compare the performance of teams whose work is underscored by good manners, trust, and civility with those of a team marked by mistrust, disrespect, and lack of consideration. For her, it's not even a contest—respect and appreciation will win every time. She also believes that effective leaders are those who are generous with their time (as we discussed in chapter 5). While they're the most heavily scheduled people in the organization, they always find the time to talk to a colleague or an employee with an urgent problem or an opportunity. They make time for others and show genuine concern. They convey, through their language and actions, that spending time with others is the most important thing a leader can do, even just 10 or 15 minutes at a time.

After stepping down from her role with the Scouts, Hesselbein founded the Frances Hesselbein Leadership Institute. As of early 2017, at the age of 101, she is still leading that organization, which is dedicated to fostering leadership grounded in "the passion to serve, the discipline to listen, the courage to question, and the spirit to include" (Frances Hesselbein Leadership Institute 2017).

2

Frances Hesselbein is a humbitious leader. She's also female. While wildly celebrated by management experts, she remains a rarity in a corporate world ruled by male leaders. Despite significant progress, women leaders still face mountainous obstacles at work. In 1995, renowned University of California, Irvine, professor Judy Rosener wrote a groundbreaking book titled *America's Competitive Secret: Women Managers.* In it, she describes American corporations and their leaders: "American institutions tend to look alike. They have similar structures and practices and similar kinds of leaders. Typically, American executives are white, male, heterosexual, and married with children. They are individualists, linear thinkers, sports fans, and usually military veterans. They also tend to be workaholics and graduates of prestigious universities. They value their families but tend to spend little time with them" (Rosener 1995, 29).

Looking at leaders of large corporations and health systems today, you can't help but feel that not much has changed since that time. While many factors have conspired to exclude women from leadership circles, the most potent is the leadership stereotypes that are widely prevalent in our workplaces. Whether they admit it or not, when most people imagine a leader, they imagine a male. In the 1970s, research uncovered a strongly held belief in organizations, referred to as *think manager–think male.* Both male and female managers believed that the traits associated with successful managers and leaders are more likely to be held by men than by women. In the 1990s, new studies revealed that while female managers no longer held these views, male managers still hung on to stereotypes (Schein 2001; Schein et al. 1996).

Despite the societal, legal, and organizational changes that have taken place since the studies were conducted, these opinions are still widely prevalent. A 2005 study conducted by the research organization Catalyst surveyed about 300 corporate leaders and asked them to rate how effective men and women are at ten essential leadership behaviors. The respondents judged male leaders to be superior to female leaders on key leadership behaviors such as problem solving, delegating, and influencing upward (Catalyst 2005). Recent reviews of the literature provide even more support for the think manager–think male paradigm: Leadership ability is still considered a prescriptive trait for men but not for women, which implies that men are expected to behave as leaders, but women aren't (Koenig et al. 2011). More recently, a field-based online experiment comparing men's and women's emotional expression revealed that women are perceived by male managers and male and female employees as lacking the qualities of emotional expression that are often associated with successful managers. Even when they have similar qualifications and capabilities, women tend to be perceived as weak leaders, whereas men are automatically presumed to be strong ones (Fischbach, Lichtenthaler, and Horstmann 2015; Grijalva et al. 2015).

3

Not only are women perceived to be less leader-like, but they also face stereotypes about how they should behave once they attain leadership positions. For example, women are generally not expected to take the initiative in projects or to speak up in discussions and meetings. In most work-related situations that require taking charge while working in a group, people tend to hold three main assumptions:

1. They expect men to be assertive, tough-minded, and aggressive, a quality sometimes referred to as *agentic*.

2. They expect women to be *communal*, which means friendly, nurturing, and accommodating.
3. They expect the person who leads the group to be agentic, not communal.

When women attempt to take charge without exhibiting agentic qualities, they're almost always ignored. However, when women assume the leadership role with an aggressive, in-your-face style, they're viewed as too masculine and unlikable, and sometimes even referred to as "bitchy" (Kramer and Harris 2014). Regardless of which approach she decides to take, a woman typically faces more obstacles than a man of equal leadership capabilities. "When a woman speaks in a professional setting, she walks a tightrope. Either she's barely heard or she's judged as too aggressive. When a man says virtually the same thing, heads nod in appreciation for his fine idea. As a result, women often decide that saying less is more," write Sheryl Sandberg, Facebook's chief operating officer, and Adam Grant, professor of management, in a recent *New York Times* series on gender roles in the workplace (Sandberg and Grant 2015).

Research backs up these views. In one study, men and women were asked to evaluate the competence of CEOs who voiced their opinions more or less frequently. When male executives spoke more frequently, they received 10 percent higher ratings on competence than their quieter peers. However, when female executives spoke more often, they were punished with 14 percent lower ratings than their less assertive peers. It turns out that "powerful women are in fact correct in assuming that they will incur backlash as a result of talking more than others" (Brescoll 2011, 622).

Moreover, women are expected to be more agreeable than men. Research conducted by the Center for Advanced Human Resource Studies (CAHRS) showed that men who are moderately disagreeable tend to earn more money than those who are agreeable. However, women who are disagreeable make as much or less than those who are agreeable. Therefore, men are expected to voice their opinions regardless of what others think and are rewarded for it in performance ratings and income, whereas women who openly express their views are perceived as deviant from their gender roles, which may result in serious economic and social penalties (CAHRS 2012).

These stereotypes can harm an organization by depriving it of valuable opinions and insights. In an experiment involving teams making strategic decisions for a bookstore, one member of the team was chosen at random to be told that the inventory system was flawed and was given information about how to improve the system. When the person with the inside knowledge who challenged the existing system was a man, team members appreciated the information and acted on it. However, when that same role was played by a woman, team members viewed her as less loyal and tended to ignore her suggestions (Brescoll 2011).

Earlier, we presented evidence that narcissism is viewed positively by others in situations of leadership emergence. This tendency appears to apply to male leaders more than female ones. Annebel de Hoogh, Deanne N. Den Hartog, and Barbora Nevicka of the University of Amsterdam studied 145 leader–subordinate pairs. They found that male subordinates rated male narcissist and nonnarcissist leaders the same way. However, when rating female leaders, they viewed female narcissists as less effective than female nonnarcissists. Women who exhibit narcissistic traits are seen as lacking stereotypically gender-appropriate qualities such as kindness and are viewed as arrogant, a quality usually associated with men (De Hoogh, Den Hartog, and Nevicka 2015).

4

In the previous chapter, we discussed the importance of generosity for leaders in terms of helping others at work. Another sizable obstacle faced by women is that they're expected to help more than men, often the type of menial work that they also do at home. However, women who help too much receive less recognition and benefit than men who engage in the same amount of help. "In keeping with deeply held gender stereotypes, we expect men to be ambitious and results-oriented, and women to be nurturing and communal. When a man offers to help, we shower him with praise and rewards. But when a woman helps, we feel less indebted. She's communal, right? She wants to be a team player. The reverse is also true. When a woman declines to help a colleague, people like her less and her career suffers. But when a man says no, he faces no backlash. A man who doesn't help is 'busy'; a woman is 'selfish,'" write Grant and Sandberg (2015). In general, women are expected to organize events, take notes at meetings, plan parties, order food, and join time-consuming committees more often than men.

Recent accounts suggest that even women who are in executive positions are expected by their male colleagues to do things like bring cupcakes for a colleague's birthday, order sandwiches for office lunches, and answer phones in the conference room (Williams and Dempsey 2014). That finding doesn't mean that men don't help. But when they do, they tend to engage in visible behaviors, such as showing up at optional meetings or speaking up when volunteers are solicited. Women, on the other hand, tend to get sucked into thankless housework activities, as well as into assisting and mentoring others behind closed doors (Eagly and Crowley 1986; Kanter 1993; Kidder 2002). Most of the help provided by women goes unnoticed—it doesn't directly translate into improved revenues. Their work also goes unrewarded by concrete promotions and salary increases. For instance, participants in a study were asked to evaluate the performance of employees who did or didn't stay late after work to help coworkers prepare for an important meeting. When a male employee stayed late and helped, he was rated 14 percent higher than a female employee who did the same. When she declined to help, a female employee was rated 12 percent lower than a male employee who declined (Heilman and Chen 2005). These double standards are real: Even when they provided identical help, men were significantly more likely to be recommended for promotions, raises, and bonuses. Women had to provide help only to be perceived equally as positively as men who didn't help.

Many of these obstacles are related to stereotypes. Another factor that prevents women from advancing as quickly as men is that they're conditioned to be less self-promoting. Leadership expert Jeffrey Pfeffer postulates that women don't use impression-management strategies as often as men do, which is part of why they're not chosen for leadership roles (Pfeffer 2015). When most women are selected for a promotion, they tend to privately question whether they're ready or deserving, whereas most men tend to think, Why did this take so long? When Pfeffer uses the term *impression management*, he describes the effort to control or influence other people's perceptions, which includes networking with high-level executives, ingratiating oneself with peers, and self-promotion. Evidence shows that many women aren't comfortable using these strategies. They believe that their high work performance and commitment will speak for themselves, and they trust the fairness of the system. Most men, on the other hand, use considerably more impression management tactics and reap the benefits in terms of promotions and rewards (Grijalva et al. 2015; Singh, Kumra, and Vinnicombe 2002).

Corinne Smith, a healthcare executive and lawyer, recently told me that she has rarely seen a woman act in a self-promoting way. "It is the way we are conditioned," she explained. "We think, 'If I just do a good job, people will notice it,' and so we don't promote our achievements" (Smith 2016). She half-joked that when most women look at the requirements of a job, if there's one aspect in which they're lacking, they decide that they're not qualified. Most men, on the other hand, look at the same requirements, and if they only meet one of them, they jump in headfirst and apply!

5

Despite the stereotypes and the confidence advantage that men seem to have, research is starting to show that women are generally more effective leaders than men, primarily because they tend to adopt a leadership style that is more suitable to the modern workplace. It is no secret that men and women tend to think and act in different ways, and these differences can be observed in their leadership styles. Typically, when a successful woman is in power, she tends to employ an interactive leadership style, whereas successful men prefer a more command-and-control style. Under the interactive style, the leader sets out to make every interaction with her subordinates positive. She encourages them to participate in decisions, she shares power and information with them, she makes them feel important, and she energizes them. In this collaborative approach, group contributions are valued as much as individual ones, and interpersonal attributes are as important as technical ones. The command-and-control model, on the other hand, is typically favored by male leaders who value clear lines of authority and who believe that decisions should be made from the top down. They view leadership as a series of transactions with subordinates and use their position and control of resources to motivate their followers. Individual performance tends to be more valued than group contributions, and fitting in with the system is a major determinant of advancement and success (Rosener 1990, 1995).

In their fascinating book *The Athena Doctrine*, authors John Gerzema and Michael D'Antonio elaborate on these differences and make a distinction between so-called masculine and feminine traits of leadership. In a study of 13 countries, Gerzema and D'Antonio first asked half of the sample of 65,000 respondents to classify 125 leadership traits as masculine, feminine, or neutral. Traits that were seen as more masculine were *dominant, arrogant, rigid, aggressive,* and *competitive*, whereas traits perceived as more feminine were *trustworthy, articulate, creative, flexible, loyal, patient,* and *cooperative* (Gerzema and D'Antonio 2013).

Gerzema and D'Antonio then presented the list of traits to the other half of the sample and asked respondents to rate the importance of these traits to leadership, success, morality, and happiness. The results showed that many of the qualities of an ideal modern leader are ones that were classified as feminine. For example, the respondents indicated a preference for an expressive style of leadership—one in which the leader shares feelings and emotions openly and honestly, a characteristic often found among women. Similarly, collaboration and sharing credit were more important than aggression and control, and being loyal topped being proud. Successful leaders were seen as those who are more intuitive and more understanding of others' feelings—those who listen, learn, and build consensus to get things done. Leaders who achieve success, have high morality, and make their employees happy are those who demonstrate connectedness, humility, openness, and flexibility. These traits were said to be personified by the Greek goddess Athena (Gerzema and D'Antonio 2013). A recent comprehensive review of 95 leadership studies on gender reached a similar conclusion. When rated by other people such as peers, bosses, subordinates, and third-party observers, female leaders were consistently perceived as more effective than male leaders. However, when self-ratings were used, male leaders viewed themselves as more effective than their female counterparts. This review confirmed that while male leaders are generally more confident, female leaders tend to be more competent (Bailey 2014; Dezsö and Ross 2012; Herring 2009; Paustian-Underdahl et al., 2014).

The world is finally starting to believe these results. Angela Merkel was appointed Germany's first woman chancellor in 2005, Erna Solberg became prime minister of Norway in 2013, and Theresa May became prime minister of Britain in 2016. In the United States, Hillary Clinton was the first female candidate of a major party in the presidential elections in 2016, although she eventually lost in a race characterized by, to say the least, significant gender tensions.

But before we get too excited about this trend of female leadership in world politics, we need to pay special attention to a concept called the *glass cliff*. While women seem to be shattering glass ceilings right and left, some experts argue that females are often chosen for leadership positions when the situation is very tough, the chances of succeeding are very low, and the males are uninterested in the job. Take, for example, the Brexit vote and the appointment of Theresa May as prime minister of Britain. Shortly after a majority of British people voted to leave the European Union, David Cameron, who had called for the referendum, announced his resignation as prime minister, while Boris Johnson, a proponent of Brexit, withdrew his bid to succeed Cameron. Facing gigantic political and economic uncertainty, the male leaders cleared the scene and left May to battle with another woman, Andrea Leadsom, for the position. The situation was seen by many as a lose–lose one for May, who faced a divided country and messy exit—a textbook glass cliff example (Bennhold 2016).

The glass cliff concept was pioneered in management studies before its use in politics. In 2003, a study compared the top 100 companies in the United Kingdom with and without women on their boards. It erroneously concluded that companies with women on their boards performed less well than all-male companies and suggested that women leaders were "wreaking havoc" on their companies' share prices (Judge 2003). Michelle Ryan and Alexander Haslam at Exeter University in Britain were skeptical about those findings. So they decided to run their own analyses on those same companies and concluded that the appointment of female directors was not, in fact, associated with a subsequent drop in company performance. More interesting, they discovered that companies that appointed female directors had consistently poor performance *before* these appointments were made, thus suggesting that female leaders were more likely to be placed in companies that were already struggling. Since that initial study, Ryan and Haslam have replicated those findings in other settings, confirming the glass cliff theory (Ryan and Haslam 2005).

6

In healthcare administration, female leaders are making significant strides, but the evidence suggests that leadership positions are still predominantly filled by men. The latest study by the American College of Healthcare Executives (ACHE) shows that only 33 percent of hospital and health system CEOs are women and that female CEOs earn on average $80,000 less than their male counterparts (ACHE 2012). Those differences are also reflected in my survey, in which 18 percent of male respondents and 5 percent of female respondents identified themselves as executives.

How did male and female respondents in the sample differ in terms of their perceptions of leadership traits? When asked to think about the one leader they had observed to be the most successful in terms of improving quality and financial outcomes in the organization and getting things done, female respondents were more likely to describe them as compassionate (41 percent of female respondents vs. 34 percent of male respondents). Male respondents were more likely to pick charismatic (26 percent of females vs. 33 percent of males) and collaborative (51 percent of females vs. 62 percent of males). On the other hand, when asked to think about the least successful leader they know, females were more likely to pick arrogant (45 percent of females vs. 35 percent of males) and inconsiderate (46 percent of females vs. 35 percent of males), while males were more likely to pick "blames others" (49 percent of females vs. 57 percent of males). (See the appendix at the end of the book for the full results.) The picture that emerges from the data is that women view successful leaders as compassionate and unsuccessful leaders as arrogant and inconsiderate. Men, on the other hand, believe that successful leaders are charismatic and collaborative, whereas unsuccessful leaders don't own up to their mistakes.

When I asked the respondents to think of individual leaders, I also urged them to specify those leaders' genders. Respondents tended to pick someone of their own gender as a successful leader: 71 percent of males picked another male, whereas 60 percent of females picked another female. When asked to compare male and female past leaders, 48 percent of *unsuccessful* male leaders were described as arrogant (vs. 36 percent of female leaders), whereas 35 percent of *unsuccessful* female leaders were described as harsh (vs. 25 percent of male leaders). Differences also emerged when respondents were asked to think of the one leader who has had a negative influence on their careers: 53 percent of *negative influence* male leaders were described as self-focused (vs. 41 percent of female leaders), and 63 percent of them were described as arrogant (vs. 42 percent of female leaders). On the other hand, only 28 percent of male leaders of *negative influence* were described as harsh (vs. 46 percent). When a man is viewed as an unsuccessful or unsupportive leader, the followers attribute much of that to his arrogance. However, when a female leader doesn't get things done or positively affect her followers' careers, it's mostly because she's perceived as harsh.

7

In 1968, Sally Hurt-Deitch was born at Providence Memorial Hospital in El Paso, Texas. Today, she is the proud CEO of that hospital and the market leader for the Hospitals of Providence network. "My mother said to me, 'You were born there and now you are back,'" she observes. "And I said, 'And if I die there, then I've gone full circle.'" She attributes many of her personal values to her upbringing in El Paso. Of those values, humility is the one of which she is most proud. "I don't like ringing my own bell, I have a real problem saying, 'Look at what I did'; I tend to say, 'Look what our team did.'" At 27, she became the youngest corporate officer ever at HCA Healthcare when she was appointed chief nursing officer at Columbia Medical Center West in El Paso (Rosin 2015). How did Sally balance personal humility with rapid career advancement?

> There are two pieces: you have to self-promote so that you can move up in your career, but you don't have to beat your chest—it should be visible through your actions. You have to champion yourself, but others can champion you too. You need to strike a balance. When I was younger I would write a lot. For example, if we are preparing for a new service line, I would put everything on paper in terms of all the preparations needed, budget, physicians, etc., and then

I would take it to my bosses and ask for their review. This is how I self-promoted in a quiet way. (Hurt-Deitch 2016)

Does she think humility has helped or hindered her career? "It is something to measure. I have been hugely successful, but could I have done more or risen faster with more self-promotion? Maybe!" (Hurt-Deitch 2016).

As a trained nurse, compassion and empathy came easily to Sally. She feels it toward her employees but also toward the patients. As she walks the hallways of her hospital, she constantly thinks to herself, "What is it like to be in that situation? How would I want to be treated?" But she's quick to note that compassion has to be accompanied by being decisive and making hard choices. "You don't want to be kind and be waffling. You can fire someone and be compassionate. I remember the first time I had to fire someone; it was hard because I was thinking, 'What I am doing to this person's life? What is the emotional and psychological impact on them and their family?' But I also thought: This person is not performing, it is more humane for them to end this quickly rather than let it linger and have others continue to talk about how lousy of a performer that person is" (Hurt-Deitch 2016). Sally doesn't believe that there are gender differences in terms of leadership styles, but she acknowledges that reactions to a certain leader's style are different for women and men. "When a man is strong and authoritative, people tend to accept it, that's how men think and talk. But when a woman behaves the same way, they have problems dealing with her and may label her as an 'ice queen' or 'bitchy.'"

Sally notes another bias in the treatment of female leaders. In some situations, married women with children aren't chosen for promotion or advancement positions because the people making the decision factor in its effects on the family. "They say, 'We've been talking about you, you are qualified and ready, but we don't know how it would affect your husband and kids!' So my reaction is, 'Are you being thoughtful or are you blowing me off because I have a family?' Let *me* make that decision!" (Hurt-Deitch 2016).

Sally's fast rise as a healthcare leader is an example that despite stereotypes and challenges, female leaders who are humbitious can achieve great things for themselves and their organizations. Let's circle back to Frances Hesselbein.

Hesselbein never thought of her gender as an obstacle; she didn't see herself as the only woman on the board with several other men. Rather, she focused on the tasks at hand and what she could bring to the table in terms of her expertise. "The management qualities that might be labeled feminine are embraced by remarkably effective women and men: leading with the power of language, cultivating relationships, building teams and structures that release the energy and potential of others, developing flexible and fluid management systems, building an organization that . . . makes the strengths of their people effective and their weaknesses irrelevant" (Hesselbein 2002, 27).

As we've highlighted in this chapter, women in leadership positions have traditionally faced unique obstacles and stereotypes that have held them back. However, their typically collaborative style, emphasizing humility, compassion, kindness, and generosity, is now more appreciated in the workplace. While these traits are feminine in a traditional sense, they're essential for both women and men who hope to thrive in the current corporate healthcare environment.

REFERENCES

American College of Healthcare Executives (ACHE). 2012. *A Comparison of the Career Attainments of Men and Women Healthcare Executives*. Published December. www.ache.org/pubs/research/2012-Gender-Report-FINAL.pdf.

Bailey, S. 2014. "Who Makes a Better Leader: A Man or a Woman?" *Forbes*. Published July 23. www.forbes.com/sites/sebastianbailey/2014/07/23/who-makes-a-better-leader-a-man-or-a-woman/#7b57b0bb9676.

Bennhold, K. 2016. "'Glass Cliff,' Not Just Ceiling, Often Impedes Women Rising in Politics." *New York Times*. Published October 5. www.nytimes.com/2016/10/05/world/europe/glass-cliff-uk -women-politics.html.

Brescoll, V. 2011. "Who Takes the Floor and Why: Gender, Power, and Volubility in Organizations." *Administrative Science Quarterly* 56 (4): 622–41.

Catalyst. 2005. "Women 'Take Care,' Men 'Take Charge': Stereotyping of U.S. Business Leaders Exposed." Published October. www.catalyst.org/system/files/Women_Take_Care_Men_Take _Charge_Stereotyping_of_U.S._Business_Leaders_Exposed.pdf.

Center for Advanced Human Resource Studies (CAHRS). 2012. "Do Nice Guys—and Gals—Really Finish Last? The Joint Effects of Sex and Agreeableness on Income." CAHRS ResearchLink No. 18. ILR School, Cornell University. Published February. http://digitalcommons.ilr.cornell.edu/cgi/viewcontent .cgi?article=1025&context=cahrs_researchlink.

De Hoogh, A., D. N. Den Hartog, and B. Nevicka. 2015. "Gender Differences in the Perceived Effectiveness of Narcissistic Leaders." *Applied Psychology* 64 (3): 473–98.

Dezsö, C., and D. Ross. 2012. "Does Female Representation in Top Management Improve Firm Performance? A Panel Data Investigation." *Strategic Management Journal* 33 (9): 1072–89.

Eagly, A. H., and M. Crowley. 1986. "Gender and Helping Behavior: A Meta-analytic Review of the Social Psychological Literature." *Psychological Bulletin* 100 (3): 283–308.

Fischbach, A., P. Lichtenthaler, and N. Horstmann. 2015. "Leadership and Gender Stereotyping of Emotions: Think Manager– Think Male." *Journal of Personnel Psychology* 14 (3): 153–62.

Frances Hesselbein Leadership Institute. 2017. "About the Institute." Accessed March 20. www.hesselbeininstitute .org/#!about_us/csgz.

Gerzema, J., and M. D'Antonio. 2013. *The Athena Doctrine: How Women (and the Men Who Think Like Them) Will Rule the Future.* San Francisco: Jossey-Bass.

Grant, A., and S. Sandberg. 2015. "Madam C.E.O., Get Me a Coffee." *New York Times.* Published February 6. www.nytimes.com/2015/02/08/opinion/sunday/sheryl-sandberg-and-adam-grant-on-women-doing-office-housework.html.

Grijalva, E., D. Newman, L. Tay, M. Donnellan, P. Harms, R. Robins, and T. Yan. 2015. "Gender Differences in Narcissism: A Meta-analytic Review." *Psychological Bulletin* 141 (2): 261–310.

Heilman, M. E., and J. J. Chen. 2005. "Same Behavior, Different Consequences: Reactions to Men's and Women's Altruistic Citizenship Behavior." *Journal of Applied Psychology* 90 (3): 431–41.

Herring, C. 2009. "Does Diversity Pay? Race, Gender, and the Business Case for Diversity." *American Sociological Review* 74 (2): 208–24.

Hesselbein, F. 2011. *My Life in Leadership.* San Francisco: Jossey-Bass.

———. 2002. *Hesselbein on Leadership.* San Francisco: Jossey-Bass.

Hurt-Deitch, S. 2016. Phone interview. September 19.

Judge, E. 2003. "Women on Board: Help or Hindrance?" *Times.* Published November 11. www.thetimes.co.uk/article/women-on-board-help-or-hindrance-2c6fnqf6fng.

Kanter, R. 1993. *Men and Women of the Corporation,* 2nd ed. New York: Basic Books.

Kidder, D. 2002. "The Influence of Gender on the Performance of Organizational Citizenship Behaviors." *Journal of Management* 28 (5): 629–48.

Koenig, A., A. Eagly, A. Mitchell, and T. Ristikari. 2011. "Are Leader Stereotypes Masculine? A Meta-analysis of Three Research Paradigms." *Psychological Bulletin* 137 (4): 616–42.

Kramer, A., and A. Harris. 2014. *Taking Control: Women, Gender Stereotypes and Impression Management*. Women's Bar Association of Illinois. Published Winter. www.luc.edu/media/lucedu /law/centers/advocacy/wil/WBAI%202014%20Taking%20 Control-%20Women%20Gender%20Stereotypes%20and%20 Impression%20Management.pdf.

Paustian-Underdahl, P., C. Samantha, L. Walker, and D. Woehr. 2014. "Gender and Perceptions of Leadership Effectiveness: A Meta-analysis of Contextual Moderators." *Journal of Applied Psychology* 99 (6): 1129–145.

Pfeffer, J. 2015. *Leadership BS: Fixing Workplaces and Careers One Truth at a Time*. New York: HarperCollins.

Rosener, J. 1995. *America's Competitive Secret: Women Managers*. New York: Oxford University Press.

———. 1990. "Ways Women Lead." *Harvard Business Review* 68 (6): 119–25.

Rosin, T. 2015. "Tenet Healthcare Names Sally Deitch CEO of Sierra Providence Health Network." *Becker's Hospital Review*. Published April 15. www.beckershospitalreview.com/hospital -executive-moves/tenet-healthcare-names-sally-deitch-ceo-of -sierra-providence-health-network.html.

Ryan, M., and A. Haslam. 2005. "The Glass Cliff: Evidence That Women Are Over-represented in Precarious Leadership Positions." *British Journal of Management* 16 (2): 81–90.

Sandberg, S., and A. Grant. 2015. "Speaking While Female." *New York Times*. January 12. www.nytimes.com/2015/01/11 /opinion/sunday/speaking-while-female.html.

Schein, V. 2001. "A Global Look at Psychological Barriers to Women's Progress in Management." *Journal of Social Issues* 57 (4): 675–88.

Schein, V., R. Mueller, T. Lituchy, and J. Liu. 1996. "Think Manager–Think Male: A Global Phenomenon?" *Journal of Organizational Behavior* 17 (1): 33–41.

Singh, V., S. Kumra, and S. Vinnicombe. 2002. "Gender and Impression Management: Playing the Promotion Game." *Journal of Business Ethics* 37 (1): 77–89.

Smith, C. 2016. Phone interview. August 29.

Williams, J., and R. Dempsey. 2014. *What Works for Women at Work: Four Patterns Working Women Need to Know.* New York: New York University Press.

CHAPTER 7

Young and Old

1

ON A HOT summer day, a dozen young, talented, ambitious computer programmers and master of business administration students arrived at IBM to complete the inaugural summer internship program Extreme Blue. They lived together in tight apartments and worked closely in small groups. Under intense pressure, they were to complete several short-term, high-impact projects. As they started their work, they quickly realized that Extreme Blue was no ordinary internship program. It was a program that emphasized, above all, humility, collaboration, and teamwork. When the Extreme Bluers finished the program at the end of the summer, they received a manual that advised them, "When you leave Extreme Blue and join another group at IBM (or any other company for that matter), we will be watching. And if we find out that you are making the program look like we are producing a bunch of arrogant wanna-bes, we will forget we ever knew you. Be ambitious. Be a leader. But do not belittle others in your pursuit of your ambitions" (Taylor 2008).

Jane Harper, the director of Internet technology and operations at IBM, is credited with starting Extreme Blue. In 1999, she dared to ask a question that no one at IBM was willing to ask: Why would really great people want to come work for us? She wondered what would entice the most gifted programmers and managers to choose her company over Google or eBay, for example. Harper predicted that the greatest people wanted to collaborate on exciting, high-impact projects in dynamic settings—which is why she created Extreme Blue.

The problem, however, was that Harper had no permission or budget to start the program. So in the first two years, she borrowed and begged for resources from other departments until the program was finally up and running (Taylor and LaBarre 2008). From those modest beginnings, Extreme Blue has now grown to a yearlong internship program hiring 250 interns and comprising more than 50 projects spread across labs in the United States, Canada, Europe, China, and India. While completing the internship, participants file hundreds of patent disclosures and transform their ideas into actual IBM products and services. About 80 percent of them end up working at IBM (IBM 2017).

The interns come to Extreme Blue with the impatience, intensity, and eagerness of all young people. They want to prove themselves and to work on meaningful projects that will make a difference. In a setting something like MTV's *Real World* meets the Manhattan Project, it would have been tempting to set those youngsters loose to fight each other aggressively for success and recognition. But a dog-eat-dog, overcompetitive environment was never part of Harper's vision. Instead, she wanted to teach the interns the value of humility and collaboration early on in their careers (Taylor 2008).

2

As an early careerist, you may be wondering why humility is so important for a future leader. In this chapter, I'll attempt to answer this question. But first, let's explore how younger people differ from other age groups in terms of humility and how that affects their leadership style.

To start with, understanding the different age groups or generations present in the workplace today is important. For the first time in the history of organizations, four distinct generations are working side by side: traditionalists (born 1900–1945), baby boomers (1946–1964), generation Xers (1965–1980), and millennials or generation Yers (1980–1999). Several factors have contributed to this phenomenon. People are living longer, and many are able to work longer. Some traditionalists and boomers are still not in a financial situation to retire, while others are supporting their generation X or millennial children.

How do these generations differ in terms of what they want at work? As of 2017, traditionalists are more than 71 years old. They're patriotic and loyal. More than half of traditionalist men are veterans. Because of their military experience, they believe that the top-down approach is the best way to get things done at work. Their management style is modeled on the military chain of command—"Leaders need to lead and troops need to follow." Baby boomers are now 52–70 years old. They're optimistic and competitive—they've had to compete with 80 million peers for everything that they've done in their lives and careers. They question authority and focus on interpersonal relations. Instead of "chain of command," they prefer "change of command." Generation Xers are 36–51 years old. They grew up witnessing many scandals and crimes, so they tend to be skeptical and self-dependent. They're most comfortable with self-command. Finally, millennials are 17–35 years old. They combine their grandparents' loyalty and optimism with their parents' skepticism, and therefore are generally realistic. They don't believe in command; rather, they prefer collaboration, communication, and participation (Knight 2014; Lancaster and Stillman 2002; Meister and Willyerd 2010).

Because this book is primarily written for the younger generation, let's focus our attention on millennials. Millennials account for more than half of the workforce today and are viewed suspiciously by the other generations at work. Bruce Tulgan is an author who studies young people in the workplace. In his book *Not Everyone Gets a Trophy*, he asked company managers what they thought about their millennial employees. Here's a collection of what they said:

- "They don't want to pay their dues and climb the ladder."
- "They walk in the door with 17 things they want to change about the company."
- "They only want to do the best tasks."
- "It's very hard to give them negative feedback without crushing their morale."
- "They walk in thinking they know more than they know."
- "They think everybody is going to get a trophy in the real world, just like they did growing up." (Tulgan 2009, 4)

It's no secret that millennials come across as entitled—their bosses and coworkers think they ask for perks before they earn them, act like spoiled brats, behave arrogantly, and think they already know everything. In job interviews, for example, most millennials ask about what the company can do for them, rather than talk about what they can do for the company. Their parents, teachers, and coaches have always focused on making them feel good about themselves and building their self-esteem. Growing up, they were told over and over, "Whatever you think, say or do, that's okay. Your feelings are true. Don't worry about how the other kids play. That's their style. You have your style. Their style is valid and your style is valid" (Tulgan 2009, 8). From this positive tolerance came the notions that everyone is a winner and everyone should get a trophy. For most millennial children, just showing up for the game was reason enough to celebrate and cheer.

The evidence also shows that school and college grades have been inflated for millennials. In the past, As were given for achievement, but now they seem to be given for effort. A recent study shows that As represent 43 percent of all letter grades given today, an increase of 28 percent since 1960 and 12 percent since 1988 (Rojstaczer and Healy 2012). I've experienced the same phenomenon with my own graduate students. For some, a B they receive from me on an assignment or exam is the first B they have gotten in their adult lives. As they sit in my office fighting back tears, I try to explain to them that an A should be awarded only for outstanding work. "But I'm outstanding! Everyone tells me that," I can see them thinking. Given that this generation grew up with soccer games where no one kept score and trophies were presented for seventh place, is it any surprise that they expect the same recognition in college?

But remembering that millennials work very hard to achieve their dreams is also important. Most have been developing their resumes practically since they were young children. In order to get ahead, millennials get involved in numerous organizations during their high school and college years and have numerous opportunities to lead others. Somewhere in that fierce competition, millennials believe they've achieved a lot, which might make older coworkers perceive them as arrogant (Alsop 2008).

In high school and college organizations, as well as at home, work is assigned based on skills, not seniority. When they get their first real job, millennials are mystified when they aren't given the lead on a certain project for which they believe they have the better skills. They don't understand some companies' requirement that you need to have seniority or experience before you can lead others (Lancaster and Stillman 2010). Because their parents treated them as equals, involved them in everything, and encouraged them to speak their minds, they expect the same from their bosses. According to Lee Caraher in *Millennials and Management*, members of the generation are accustomed to constant acknowledgment and appreciation, which makes it hard for people who work with them to keep up with those expectations (Caraher 2015).

In the workplace, it appears that millennials want constant recognition for what managers of other generations consider regular work. I spoke with Amelie Karam, an expert on millennial issues and a millennial herself, who argues that the notion of self-absorbed millennials is largely a stereotype. She offers a different perspective: "We were raised by parents and teachers that focused on us as individuals, that made us feel special. As a result, we believe that we are special, but also that every person is special. Everyone is unique, and we accept their point of view. This is not arrogance, it is just a different take on humility" (Karam 2016). Millennials aren't arrogant in the sense that they think they're better than everyone else. Rather, they truly believe that they bring special skills and capabilities to the table, and that everyone else does too.

3

To better comprehend millennials' leadership styles, a good place to start is what they want from their bosses. Millennials seek leaders who will help them navigate their career paths, give them straight feedback, are comfortable with flexible schedules, sponsor them for development programs, and mentor and coach them (Meister and Willyerd 2010). They want their bosses to give them advice and guidance and share stories about mistakes they've made. But they don't necessarily want to follow in the footsteps of their bosses— they're more interested in setting their own paths. What millennials really want is what experts refer to as *in loco parentis* bosses—a Latin term that means "in the place of a parent." They want their bosses to show them that they care, just as their parents did. For example, one millennial Tulgan interviewed wanted his boss to be someone "who know(s) who I am and what I'm doing, and who seems to care. I've had bosses who didn't even know my name. But right now I'm working for this woman who is very busy, but she really connects with me, eye-to-eye kind of, asks me questions and really listens. She's taught me a lot already" (Tulgan 2009, 61). Amelie agrees with this notion and notes that millennials don't want to be CEOs tomorrow because they know that they're not ready. In her research, she has found that about 80 percent of millennials prefer gradually stepping into a leadership role over moving immediately. What they want is to be mentored and guided by their bosses in order to prepare themselves for the upcoming challenges in their careers.

"We don't want it to be handed to us, we want to work hard to get it, but we need support along the way," she explains (Karam 2016).

If a mentor or a coach is their preferred boss, how do millennials actually behave when in a leadership position themselves? Little research has examined how generations differ in terms of leadership styles, but the closest is research on the connection between age and leadership. In a study of more than 400 leaders and managers in the United Kingdom, younger managers were found to be less consultative than their older counterparts. They were also more likely to promote themselves, whereas older ones tended to devote their time to helping others develop their careers. The study explained that younger managers may think that they already know what's best for their units and consider consultation unnecessary or a waste of time. They also may be more willing to take risks and try new approaches. On the other hand, older managers involve employees in order to get their buy-in and support for decisions (Oshagbemi 2004).

In another study, the transformational leadership style of 56 leaders was evaluated by their followers. Transformational leadership refers to behaviors such as inspirational motivation (talking optimistically about the future), idealized influence (instilling pride in others for being associated with the leader), individualized consideration (spending time teaching and coaching), and intellectual stimulation (reexamining critical assumptions to question whether they're appropriate). The results showed that people older than 46 are rated the highest for overall transformational leadership, whereas the lowest ratings for intellectual stimulation and individualized consideration are given to the 36–45 age group (Barbuto et al. 2007).

Similarly, a report by the Management Research Group examined two specific aspects of leadership: cooperation and empathy. It defines cooperation as accommodating the needs and interests of others by being willing to defer working on one's own objectives in order to assist colleagues with theirs, whereas empathy refers to demonstrating an active concern for people and their needs by forming close and supportive relationships with them. The participants consisted of 640 younger (25–35 years) and 640 older (45–55 years) unit and department managers who completed 360-degree evaluations. These types of evaluations ask leaders to rate themselves and then ask their bosses, colleagues, and subordinates to rate them as well. Because 360-degree evaluations are comprehensive, they're considered the closest thing to the truth in terms of the actual style of a certain leader. The findings indicate that older managers receive higher ratings than younger ones on cooperation by their bosses and their peers. They're also rated higher on empathy by their bosses, peers, and direct reports (Kabacoff and Stoffey 2001).

A more recent study of Indian managers and employees in a sugar factory concluded that leaders start early in their careers with an autocratic leadership style and then move toward a democratic style in middle age; at the later stages, they use a laissez-faire style. It's possible that with growing knowledge and experience, leaders become more capable of understanding others and therefore tend to become more flexible and less assertive, feeling less need to exert authority on others (Kotur and Anbazhagan 2014). These studies suggest that younger employees want an understanding boss, but they tend to be less involved with their team once they're placed in a leadership position.

Noting that these results cannot be generalized to all organizations and settings is important, as the culture of the organization may send powerful messages to millennials about how to behave. "As managers, we are very collaborative and inclusive," says Amelie, the generational expert. "However, when working in an organization where the culture is about survival of the fittest, we may feel that it is not safe for us to help others" (Karam 2016). The IBM internship culture was built around collaboration and humility, but other organizations don't necessarily share these values and principles.

4

To better understand young people's views on leadership in healthcare organizations, let's turn to the results of my survey. I categorized the respondents into three age groups: 18–34 years old (representing millennials, more or less), 35–54 years old (representing generation X), and 55–74 years old (representing baby boomers). (See the appendix at the end of the book for the complete results.) First, how do the age groups differ in terms of the traits of leaders who have had a positive influence on their careers? For the younger generation, the top five traits are *accountable, compassionate, kind, humble,* and *generous.* While the other age groups also chose those first three traits, *humble* and *generous* didn't make it in the top five for either one of them. As for leaders who are perceived to be successful in terms of improving financial and quality outcomes in the organization, the top five traits for millennials were *accountable, collaborative, ambitious, holds others accountable,* and *generous.* Whereas *accountable, collaborative,* and *holds others accountable* were also in the top five for generation Xers and baby boomers, *ambitious* and *generous* were highly ranked only by millennials. The three generations more or less agreed on the top five traits of leaders with a negative influence or who were unsuccessful. The results suggest that millennials appreciate humility and generosity more in leaders who can help them in their own personal development, whereas they value ambition and generosity more in successful leaders.

5

The finding that millennials appreciate humility more than the other generations is somewhat surprising, given the perception that they're not humble themselves. However, millennials are outgoing and gregarious, which may affect their perception by others. When we examined humility in chapter 2, I noted that we should consider extraversion and introversion, as these personality types can influence leadership style. Years of research have shown that millennials are in fact more extraverted than older generations, which doesn't make them appear humble (Donnellan and Lucas 2008; Lehmann et al. 2013).

We've also established that millennials value humility in their leaders, and think of themselves as humble and special at the same time. But is humility a necessary condition for success for early careerists or is it a hindrance? Some experts and researchers think that humility can actually derail young leaders. Examining the evidence for Level 5 leaders (which we discussed in previous chapters), leadership thinker and writer Jeffrey Pfeffer is very skeptical that humility and modesty can help young leaders get to the top. He notes that Collins assessed leadership qualities of people already in CEO positions but didn't examine how they got there in the first place (Pfeffer 2015).

A similar conclusion was reached in the *Harvard Business Review* article "Why Bossy Is Better for Rookie Managers," which reports on the results of two experiments (Sauer 2012). First, business school students watched video clips of actors portraying young, inexperienced team leaders and were asked to rate their effectiveness on a 1–7 scale. Leaders who just told others what to do got an average rating of 4.25, whereas those who solicited opinions of their team members got a rating of 3.55. Second, undergraduate students were placed in teams working on a complex computer-based task. They were tasked with solving problems with the fewest possible clicks of the mouse. Leaders were ranked by their team members on confidence and effectiveness, while team performance was measured by the total number of clicks needed to solve a problem. Leaders who adopted a directive approach received higher ratings in terms of both confidence and effectiveness than those who took a participative approach. Moreover, teams with directive leaders needed an average of 108 clicks to solve a problem, whereas those with participative leaders needed about 126 clicks. Study author Stephen Sauer offers the following explanation:

> If these results seem counterintuitive, imagine this: You're on an experienced team that gets an unfamiliar leader. You look for clues about his status—How old is he? How does he dress? Where did he train?—and form an assessment

accordingly. If he seems to be a lightweight, you'll probably resist his attempts to influence you. And if he asks
for your input, chances are even greater that you'll view
him as lacking in competence. But if he's directive and
assertive, you'll take that as confidence, and you'll come to
see him as more able than you first thought. His perceived
capabilities will rise. (Sauer 2012)

The results suggest that when a younger manager assumes a leadership position, she's better off setting her agenda, establishing a
clear direction, and telling people exactly what to do. Humility and
collaboration, it seems, can wait till later, when the leader is finally
viewed as experienced and knowledgeable. While there is definitely
some wisdom in this perspective, in the next few sections I'll provide
evidence that shows that the reality may be a bit different.

6

Imagine a group of new healthcare administration recruits at a large
health system, dressed to the nines, leather folders in one hand and
smartphones in the other. How likely are these up-and-comers to
share some of the foundations of humility that we discussed in
chapter 2, such as fallibility, vulnerability, transparency, inadequacy,
and interdependency? If we're honest, very unlikely. Understanding why these attributes aren't seen as leading to advancement and
success is easy. Showing weaknesses, admitting mistakes, and asking
for help aren't exactly what gets early careerists noticed. "Particularly in the United States and throughout much of the Western
industrialized world, the attributes that get leaders (especially young
leaders) noticed are attributes of independence, determination,
quick thinking, and a pioneering spirit, which ultimately form
the backbone of a Darwinian selection process that separates high
potential leaders from their peers," note leadership development
experts Erik Hoekstra, Antony Bell, and Scott Peterson (2008, 81).

Acting confident, focusing on one's self only, and tooting one's own horn are seen by many young people as necessary in order to strive and advance in an overly competitive world.

In 2008, when Jean Twenge and colleagues published a study documenting the rise in narcissism among the younger generation, they faced a significant reaction from young people who insisted that narcissism was crucial for competing for prestigious universities and high-paying jobs. In their subsequent book, titled *The Narcissism Epidemic*, Twenge and coauthor Keith Campbell (2009) document the prevalent attitude among young people that they need to do whatever it takes to get ahead. For example, one university student wrote of the narcissism study results, "The people conducting this research didn't have to deal with the amount of competition we face daily. We have to be confident and focused on ourselves in order to succeed. So if our generation seems a little more obsessed with 'Me' than those before us, it is not our fault" (Twenge and Campbell 2009, 41). Another student wrote a related column in her university's newspaper, stating, "Today's college students have more pressure and stress put on them than in past years. The way we're able to meet and exceed the challenges we face is by believing in ourselves. Feeling special is a great form of motivation" (Twenge and Campbell 2009, 41). A 27-year-old wrote in the comments section of the *New York Times*: "Aren't self-confidence and belief in oneself basic requirements for success in one's personal and professional life? If that's the definition of a narcissist, proud to be one. And a successful one at that ☺" (Twenge and Campbell 2009, 41).

In the face of this criticism, Twenge and Campbell argue that these young people are wrong in assuming that self-confidence, even narcissism, can lead them to success. The researchers present study after study that have found that this popular belief is simply not true. For example, college students who have inflated views of themselves tend to receive poorer grades and are more likely to drop out. Their overconfidence backfires because they aren't good at taking criticism and learning from their mistakes. They tend to think that they already know it all, a phenomenon that psychologists call *overclaiming*.

In one study, for instance, people were asked to answer 150 questions, including 30 questions that the authors made up specifically for the test. Some of these questions related to the jazz great Milton Silus, the painter John Kormat, and the Treaty of Monticello. Narcissists pretended to know everything about these characters and events, even the ones that don't actually exist (Twenge and Campbell 2009). While Twenge and Campbell clearly show that overconfidence and narcissism do not, in fact, lead to success, they recognize that some form of self-promotion is necessary today for young people. They posit that "self-promotion is more necessary now than it once was. When you switch jobs more often, you have to know how to polish your résumé and sound good in an interview. With college admissions more competitive, students must 'package themselves' to get in." But they also warn that it's possible to be self-promoting when necessary without being completely narcissistic. In that sense, self-promotion is only one tool in the toolbox, something useful under specific circumstances but not an obsessive activity that defines one's personality (Twenge and Campbell 2009, 51).

7

To get some clarity on the issues of humility, narcissism, and self-promotion among early careerists, I turned to two respected healthcare leaders at two stages of their careers: a midcareer, seasoned executive, and an up-and-comer. Marc Strode is the current CEO of Methodist Stone Oak Hospital in San Antonio, a 140-bed hospital that was recently ranked sixth in the country on quality of care by *Hospital Compare*. Marc started his career in 1998 as a resident at Methodist Hospital. His preceptor was Jim Scoggin, the CEO of Methodist Hospital at the time. "Jim was exhibit A in humility," says Marc. "He taught me how important it is to be humble to create the right platform to develop relationships that are built on mutual respect between two human beings." Marc truly believes that humility is crucial for young healthcare administrators:

> The minute you set foot in the hospital on the first day of your residency, people start judging you, to determine whether you are self-entitled or not. Jim would never have allowed me to be self-entitled, and I don't allow our residents to be that way. As a resident and early careerist, it is very important to manage your reputation. Don't get too far ahead of yourself, thinking I can be CEO in no time. At this stage in your career, the train can quickly derail if you are seen as a know-it-all, self-entitled, too full of yourself just because you've been to graduate school. (Strode 2016)

"How can you balance humility with being noticed and chosen for promotion and career development?" I asked Marc. "My approach is to build the relationships first, which leads to opportunities for advancement. If you don't do that, you start to press, you ask 'how do I make my mark?' Instead, you should start by getting to know the organization, the people. And you say to yourself: 'I will learn first by listening and observing, learn from others, show respect to the team. These people have been here much longer than me, they know more than I do, and they could[n't] care less that I have a master's" (Strode 2016).

An important factor in all of that is the work ethic. In Marc's experience, it's the glue that binds relationships with advancement. "Work ethic is about rolling your sleeves and working side by side with the dishwasher. Sure, one day you might be their boss's boss, but for now they have seniority over you and you respect their trade, their craft, and appreciate there's a lot to learn from them. At the end of the day, no one on the team is more important than anyone else. If you are going to lead in healthcare and be successful at it, you must take that approach" (Strode 2016).

Enrique Gallegos offers a similar perspective. Graduating from his master of health administration class in 2006, Enrique climbed the leadership ladder in record time—he is now CEO of the Laredo Medical Center, a 326-bed hospital located in south Texas near the Mexican border. When he first started in his career, he didn't need anyone to remind him of his own limitations.

> As a resident, I came in with an inquisitive mind, I made sure to demonstrate humility by showing deference and respect to others. In your first leadership role, it's important to recognize that the people reporting to you are the experts and you are not, particularly if you have technical departments such as the laboratory or respiratory therapy. Some of the directors in those departments have been at the hospital longer than you have been alive. You don't come in with the attitude "I have an MHA, I know everything!" You give people their place, you draw on their expertise. Your role is support and facilitation; you try to help them with career advancement. (Gallegos 2016)

As for getting noticed and promoted, Enrique emphasizes the importance of volunteering for all types of projects (even nonglamorous ones) and taking advantage of what he calls *pivotal opportunities*. He explains:

> You give credit to others where credit is due, but when you are tasked with a major imperative, you should recognize that it is a golden opportunity to showcase your skills and for you to be known as a capable and committed member of the team. For example, after I finished my residency, the compliance officer position became vacant. I didn't aspire to be the compliance officer, and quite honestly, wasn't after a title. However, my mentor told me it would be a wonderful opportunity and that I would add it to my current responsibilities as assistant administrator. I followed his

advice and took the position, even though I didn't have any knowledge or experience in compliance. I dedicated the necessary time to learn it and was excited about the opportunity to report directly to the CEO, as it was a great way to get noticed. When you are starting out and trying to make a name for yourself, you need to recognize you are competing with others for the limelight, so you need to come across as capable and as having the leadership skills needed to contribute to the organization's mission. You get noticed by the results that you deliver, but also by volunteering for different projects. When you are not tapped, you should volunteer, even if it is for a project that is not very glamorous, but may have a big impact. (Gallegos 2016)

8

Healthcare leaders truly believe that young people can be successful without demanding credit or puffing themselves up. Jane Harper from IBM, who created Extreme Blue, agrees: "I always urge new people not to worry about 'getting credit or taking credit' for great work. If they're making bold moves, and developing good relationships, they will get more opportunities to grow and succeed. Don't waste energy on worrying about whether everything you do gets noticed. It does" (Taylor 2008).

Confidence, determination, assertiveness, and independence are all important in the struggle to be noticed and promoted. But too often, these attributes define early leadership potential, and—when left unchecked—they can lead to derailment later on in a career. When leaders start to enjoy achievement and success, promotions and accolades are thrown at them. Before long, they start reading and believing their own press clippings and success goes to their heads. They start feeling special and attributing their success exclusively to their unique talent. Once they buy into this lie, they believe that others think of them as special and, most dangerously, as perfect.

When faced with complex challenges, they tell themselves things such as, "Always look like everything is under control," "Don't let them see you sweat," and "Take extreme risks—that's what leaders do." By not admitting their weaknesses, not learning from their mistakes, and not involving others in decision making, they set themselves up for failure as leaders.

Jane Harper is very humble herself. She doesn't think she has any special talent other than the ability to find talented individuals and help them develop their own abilities. She strongly believes that humility, coupled with ambition, can lead to achievement. She has coined the term *humbition* (which I've used throughout this book): the subtle blend of humility and ambition that drives the most successful leaders. These leaders are ambitious, constantly seeking success, but when it finally arrives, they're humbled. They recognize that they owe much of their achievements to other people, to luck, to timing, and to many other factors. They're gracious and open to others' ideas, because they understand their own limitations (Taylor 2008).

The take-home message for young careerists is that when you're just starting as an intern or employee, you should show humility—but promote yourself enough through your actions to be noticed. When you take on a leadership position, you need to show confidence and directedness, but beware of being perceived as a whippersnapper.

REFERENCES

Alsop, R. 2008. *The Trophy Kids Grow Up: How the Millennial Generation Is Shaking Up the Workplace.* San Francisco: Jossey-Bass.

Barbuto, J. E., Jr., S. Fritz, G. S. Matkin, and D. B. Marx. 2007. "Effects of Gender, Education, and Age upon Leaders' Use of Influence Tactics and Full Range Leadership Behaviors." *Sex Roles* 56: 71–83.

Caraher, L. 2015. *Millennials and Management: The Essential Guide to Making It Work at Work*. Brookline, MA: Bibliomotion.

Donnellan, M. B., and R. E. Lucas. 2008. "Age Differences in the Big Five Across the Life Span: Evidence from Two National Samples." *Psychology and Aging* 23 (3): 558–66.

Gallegos, E. 2016. Phone interview. September 30.

Hoekstra, E., A. Bell, and S. R. Peterson. 2008. "Humility in Leadership: Abandoning the Pursuit of Unattainable Perfection." In *Executive Ethics: Ethical Dilemmas and Challenges for the C-Suite*, edited by S. A. Quatro and R. R. Sims, 79–96. Greenwich, CT: Information Age Publishing.

IBM. 2017. "Extreme Blue." Accessed March 24. www-01.ibm.com/employment/us/extremeblue/.

Kabacoff, R., and R. Stoffey. 2001. "Age Differences in Organizational Leadership." Paper presented at the Sixteenth Annual Convention of the Society for Industrial and Organizational Psychology, San Diego, CA, April 27.

Karam, A. 2016. Personal interview. September 30.

Knight, R. 2014. "Managing People from Five Generations." *Harvard Business Review*. Published September 25. https://hbr.org/2014/09/managing-people-from-5-generations.

Kotur, B. R., and S. Anbazhagan. 2014. "The Influence of Age and Gender on the Leadership Styles." *IOSR Journal of Business and Management* 16 (1): 30–36.

Lancaster, L., and D. Stillman. 2010. *The M-factor: How the Millennial Generation Is Rocking the Workplace*. New York: Harper Business.

———. 2002. *When Generations Collide: Who They Are, Why They Clash, How to Solve the Generational Puzzle at Work*. New York: HarperCollins.

Lehmann, R., J. A. Denissen, M. Allemand, and L. Penke. 2013. "Age and Gender Differences in Motivational Manifestations of the Big Five from Age 16 to 60." *Developmental Psychology* 49 (2): 365–83.

Meister, J. C., and K. Willyerd. 2010. "Mentoring Millennials." *Harvard Business Review*. Published May. https://hbr.org/2010/05/mentoring-millennials.

Oshagbemi, T. 2004. "Age Influences on the Leadership Styles and Behavior of Managers." *Employee Relations* 26 (1): 14–29.

Pfeffer, J. 2015. *Leadership BS: Fixing Workplaces and Careers One Truth at a Time*. New York: Harper Business.

Rojstaczer, S., and C. Healy. 2012. "Where A Is Ordinary: The Evolution of American College and University Grading, 1940–2009." *Teachers College Record* 114 (7). www.gradeinflation.com/tcr2012grading.pdf.

Sauer, S. J. 2012. "Why Bossy Is Better for Rookie Managers." *Harvard Business Review*. Published May. https://hbr.org/2012/05/why-bossy-is-better-for-rookie-managers.

Strode, M. 2016. Personal interview. September 26.

Taylor, B. 2008. "On the 'Battle for Talent' and the Power of 'Humbition.'" *Harvard Business Review*. Published February 27. https://hbr.org/2008/02/on-the-battle-for-talent-and-t.

Taylor, W. C., and P. G. LaBarre. 2008. *Mavericks at Work: Why the Most Original Minds in Business Win*. New York: HarperCollins.

Tulgan, B. 2009. *Not Everyone Gets a Trophy*. San Francisco: Jossey-Bass.

Twenge, J. M., and W. K. Campbell. 2009. *The Narcissism Epidemic: Living in the Age of Entitlement*. New York: Atria Paperback.

Twenge, J. M., S. Konrath, J. D. Foster, W. K. Campbell, and B. J. Bushman. 2008. "Egos Inflating over Time: A Cross-temporal Meta-analysis of the Narcissistic Personality Inventory." *Journal of Personality* 76 (4): 875–901.

CHAPTER 8

Nature and Nurture

1

At 27, Benjamin Franklin embarked on an ambitious project to achieve "moral perfection." He identified 12 virtues that he wanted to master. These consist of the following, in his own words:

1. Temperance: Eat not to dullness; drink not to elevation.
2. Silence: Speak not but what may benefit others or yourself; avoid trifling conversation.
3. Order: Let all your things have their places; let each part of your business have its time.
4. Resolution: Resolve to perform what you ought; perform without fail what you resolve.
5. Frugality: Make no expense but to do good to others or yourself, i.e., waste nothing.
6. Industry: Lose no time; be always employed in something useful; cut off all unnecessary actions.
7. Sincerity: Use no hurtful deceit; think innocently and justly, and, if you speak, speak accordingly.
8. Justice: Wrong none by doing injuries or omitting the benefits that are your duty.
9. Moderation: Avoid extremes; forbear resenting injuries so much as you think they deserve.

10. Cleanliness: Tolerate no uncleanliness in body, clothes, or habitation.
11. Tranquility: Be not disturbed at trifles, or at accidents common or unavoidable.
12. Chastity: Rarely use venery but for health or offspring, never to dullness, weakness, or the injury of your own or another's peace or reputation. (Eliot 2010, 79)

When Franklin asked a Quaker friend to look over the list, the man suggested that he should add another virtue: *humility*. He told Franklin that he was "generally thought proud" and "overbearing and rather insolent" and gave him several examples in which he had demonstrated that pride (Campbell 1999, 141). Convinced by those arguments, Franklin made humility, which he understood as imitating Jesus and Socrates, his thirteenth virtue. He then put together a detailed schedule to work on the 13 virtues one at a time over 13 weeks, while repeating the cycle four times per year. In order to track his progress, he created a record book and made a black mark each time he failed to exhibit a virtue on which he was working. His daily schedule consisted of seven hours for sleep, eight hours for work, and nine hours for planning, reviewing, and reflecting on his virtues, as well as eating, relaxing, and reading (Bobb 2013).

To become more humble, Franklin had a meticulous plan to change what he said and how he behaved with others:

I made it a rule to forbear all direct contradiction to the sentiments of others, and all positive assertion of my own. I even forbid myself, agreeably to the old laws of our Junto, the use of every word or expression in the language that imported a fixed opinion, such as certainly, undoubtedly, etc., and I adopted, instead of them, I conceive, I apprehend, or I imagine a thing to be so or so, or it so appears to me at present. When another asserted something that I thought an error, I denied myself the pleasure of contradicting him abruptly and of showing immediately some absurdity in his proposition; and in answering, I began by observing that in certain cases or circumstances his opinion would be right, but in the present case there appeared or seemed to me some difference, etc. I soon found the advantage of this change in my manner; the conversations I engaged in went on more pleasantly. (Eliot 2010, 87)

But of all the virtues that he worked on, Franklin admitted that humility proved to be the most difficult for him. "In reality, there is, perhaps, no one of our natural passions so hard to subdue as pride. Disguise it, struggle with it, beat it down, stifle it, mortify it as much as one pleases, it is still alive, and will every now and then peep out and show itself" (Campbell 1999, 141). No matter how hard he tried, he couldn't get over his pride and ego.

More than 200 years later, scholars tend to agree with this view. June Price Tangney, a researcher who studies humility, notes that over time, humans have developed a reflexive tendency to protect and defend themselves in order to survive, which runs counter to being humble. Humility, therefore, tends to be very rare among people today (Tangney 2000). Similarly, Everett Worthington, a professor and clinical psychologist who is considered an authority on virtues, agrees that reaching humility is extremely hard. In his remarkable book *Humility: The Quiet Virtue*, he notes that "perhaps humility is not something we can systematically learn in some five-step program. Perhaps the opposite of humility—self-focus—is too ingrained in our nature" (Worthington 2007, 51).

The evidence that we've examined so far suggests that humility, compassion, kindness, and generosity are related to the leaders' personality, upbringing, and early career experiences. In this final chapter, we discuss whether these traits can be trained for and taught and how self-centered leaders can change and improve. We also explore specific humility and compassion training programs and evaluate their effectiveness.

When Jim Collins was working on *Good to Great*, he was invited to talk to a group of senior executives. He shared his finding about Level 5 leaders: Out of 1,435 companies he and his team studied, only 11 made the transition from good to great. All of these were led by Level 5 leaders—that is, CEOs who had a paradoxical blend of humility and fierce determination. A woman in the audience, a recently appointed CEO, raised her hand with concern and admitted, "I am disturbed because when I look in the mirror, I know that I'm not a Level 5, not yet anyway. Part of the reason I got this job is because of my ego drives." She then proceeded to ask the million-dollar question: "Can you learn to become a Level 5?" (Collins 2001, 35).

Collins hypothesizes that there are two categories of people: those who have the seeds of Level 5 leadership and those who don't. He argues that the vast majority of people have the potential to evolve to that level, though their innate abilities may be forgotten or underused. When triggered by a specific person or event, they begin to progress. They might begin self-reflecting or engage in conscious personal development. They may encounter a great coach, a mentor, or a Level 5 leader, or they may undergo a significant life experience. For example, Darwin Smith, the Level 5 leader of Kimberly Clark whom we met in chapter 2, learned that he had throat cancer around the same time he became CEO. The doctors told him that he had one year to live at most. He underwent radiation treatment, regained his health, and went on to serve as a successful CEO for 20 years (Barboza 1995).

While not everyone needs to be diagnosed with cancer in order to start this kind of transformation, major life events may force leaders to introspect and think about the deeper meanings of their work and their lives. The second category of people—those who don't have the seed for Level 5—are a minority. Collins describes them as "people who could never in a million years bring themselves to subjugate their egoistic needs to the greater ambition of building something larger and more lasting than themselves. For these people, work will always be first and foremost about what they *get*—fame, fortune, adulation, power, whatever—not what they *build*, create, and contribute." Achieving Level 5 leadership is almost impossible for this type (Collins 2001, 36).

What about the rest of us, who aren't egomaniacs but who know that we need to become more humble—is there a clearly defined path? Collins admits that he doesn't have a list of steps that leaders can follow, because no robust research on the topic exists. He remarks that "a '10-Step List to Level 5' would trivialize the concept" (Collins 2001, 38). Rather, he suggests that leaders who are serious about reaching Level 5 leadership should practice the other concepts that have helped the companies he studied achieve greatness, given the symbiotic relationship that exists between these principles and Level 5 leadership.

For example, leaders should start by focusing on the people they want on their team before deciding on their vision ("First who, then what"). They should simplify their complex world into a single, organizing idea that unifies, organizes, and guides all their decisions ("Be a hedgehog, not a fox"). Then, through disciplined action, they should decide what they're going to stop doing in addition to what they're going to start doing ("The stop-doing list"). While there is no guarantee that practicing these principles actually leads to Level 5 leadership, Collins argues that it can provide a tangible place to begin (Collins 2001). It appears then that achieving Level 5 leadership, and gaining the humility that it requires, is a complex process that can't be reduced to simple steps. It requires countless hours of self-reflection and slow behavioral change, which may be supported by coaching.

3

I've been a university professor for 14 years. Since I started, students have come to me for advice about their careers and professional development. Some need help with their interviewing skills, while others seek clarity in choosing the right administrative residency. Recent graduates need direction about picking their first jobs or dealing with a difficult boss. I've always tried to listen attentively, ask questions, and provide advice when needed. Little did I know that I've actually been coaching. A couple years ago, I started learning more about executive coaching, in part because I felt the need to go beyond common sense and intuition when helping others and to acquire some tools and skills that can maximize the potential from those interactions. I completed a certification in executive coaching, as well as programs in assessments, including emotional intelligence and personality testing. During 2016, I formally coached about 20 senior and midlevel executives.

"What is coaching?" many people ask me. *Coaching* is helping executives identify gaps between where they are and where they need to be, inspiring more intentional thinking and behavioral changes than they would have required of themselves. It's about creating a safe environment in which people see themselves more clearly (Arruda 2014). In short, the executive coach is a thought partner who can help busy executives find the time and space to think deeply about important issues. For example, when faced with a specific problem at work, the executive can seek the coach's help in order to formulate goals in dealing with that problem, identify the options available to achieve those goals, anticipate and better negotiate obstacles that might prevent him from reaching the goals, and commit to specific short-term and long-term actions and changes to sustain those goals. Using a well-thought-out plan, the coach holds the executive accountable for those actions and changes. Many experts believe that executive coaching has remarkable potential to help leaders make progress toward humility and compassion.

Marshall Goldsmith is one of the most famous executive coaches of our time. He specializes in working with highly successful people to focus on little flaws that prevent them from becoming even more successful. In his widely popular book *What Got You Here Won't Get You There* (2007)—the bible of executive coaching—he explains that successful people have important beliefs and habits that have helped them become successful. Ironically, those same beliefs and habits stand in the way of changing behavior and achieving more success. In other words, what got them to be successful won't get them to become more successful. Goldsmith identifies about 20 habits that hold successful people back. Many of those habits are directly related to the issues in this book and are the opposite of behaviors that make a Level 5 leader.

Goldsmith argues that most successful people win too much. After all, that's how they became successful. However, that addiction to winning becomes harmful when it leads to the need to win at all costs and in all situations—"When it matters, when it doesn't, and when it's totally beside the point" (Goldsmith 2007, 40). They also constantly need to add value and display an overwhelming desire to give their two cents in every discussion. For example, when a subordinate comes to the successful executive with a new idea that she's excited about, the executive can't help but say, "I can make your idea much better." By doing that, Goldsmith explains, the executive may improve the idea by 5 percent but will definitely decrease the motivation of the subordinate to implement the idea by 50 percent.

Many successful people also like to pass judgment and have a need to rate others and impose their own standards. They're also accustomed to making destructive comments, which include needless sarcasm and cutting remarks that they think make them sound sharp and witty. They start most of their sentences with "no," "but," or "however." These negative qualifiers are their way of telling everyone, "I'm right and you're wrong." They constantly need to tell the world how smart they are.

Some highly successful people also like to withhold information and refuse to share important details in order to maintain an advantage over others. This tendency includes not answering e-mails or returning phone calls, or providing partial explanations. Others fail to give proper recognition or credit and even claim credit when they don't deserve it. When things don't go their way, they make excuses and deflect blame from themselves and onto other people and events. Many also refuse to express regret; they're unable to take responsibility for their actions, admit that they're wrong, or recognize how their actions affect others. Finally, many successful people don't listen, thus demonstrating the most passive-aggressive form of disrespect for their colleagues and coworkers (Goldsmith 2007).

Goldsmith explains that most successful leaders have only a few, at most, of these bad habits. His approach in helping people get rid of a habit focuses first on making them realize that they *have* the habit. He starts by conducting a 360-degree evaluation for each executive by collecting input from his coworkers (boss, subordinates, colleagues) and family members. Once the feedback is collected and the bad habits are confirmed, he relates them to the executive and holds him accountable by having him apologize to others for those behaviors. He then asks him to announce to others that he's working on changing and has him commit to following up on a periodic basis to ask them about his progress (Goldsmith 2007).

One day, Goldsmith was called to work with an investment banker, a rising star he calls Mike. According to Goldsmith (2017), Mike "could have inspired the Gordon Gekko character," in reference to the callous and deceiving personality played by Michael Douglas in the movie *Wall Street*. Goldsmith tells the story of how he worked to coach Mike:

> Mike's score for treating colleagues with respect was dismal; in fact, out of 1,000 managers rated, he was dead last! But Mike put up astounding numbers with his trades. His profit contribution was so vast that the CEO promoted him into management. This should have been the apex of Mike's young career.
>
> Instead, it exposed his bad side. The firm's leaders, who had been insulated from Mike's behavior, were suddenly getting a first-hand dose of his "lead, follow, or get out of my way" style. In meetings, they saw that there was often no checkpoint between Mike's brain and mouth.

He was surly and offensive to everyone, even to the CEO, who called me in to "help him change now." When I met Mike, I noticed his delight in his success. He was making more than $4 million a year, so professional validation was coursing through his veins like jet fuel. I knew that breaking through to Mike by challenging his performance would be tough. He was delivering results, and he knew it.

So I told him, "I can't help you make more money. But let's talk about your ego. How do you treat people at home?"

Mike insisted that he was a great husband and father. "I don't bring my work home," he assured me. "I'm a warrior on Wall Street but a pussycat at home."

"Is your wife home right now?"

"Yes," he said.

"Why don't you call her and see how different she thinks you are at home?" He called his wife. She agreed that Mike was a jerk at home, too. Then he got his two kids on the line, and they agreed with their mother.

"I'm beginning to see a pattern here," I said. "Do you really want to have a funeral that no one attends other than for business reasons?" Mike looked stricken. "They're going to fire me if I don't make my numbers, aren't they?" he asked.

"Not only are they going to fire you," I said, "but several people will be dancing in the halls when you go." Mike reflected on that, and said, "I'm going to change, and the reason has nothing to do with money or with this firm. I have two sons, and if they were receiving this feedback from you in 20 years, I'd be ashamed to be their father." Within a year, Mike's scores on his treatment of people shot up past the 50th percentile, above an already high company norm. He probably deserved even better, since he started so far down in the ditch. He also doubled his income. (Goldsmith 2017)

When leaders want to know how their behavior comes across to their colleagues, Goldsmith advises them to stop looking in the mirror to admire themselves. Instead, he asks them to let their colleagues hold the mirror for them and tell them what they see. He contends that, just like Mike, anyone can change if he has an important enough reason to do so. In a 2013 *Harvard Business Review* article, consultants John Dame and Jeffrey Gedmin echo Goldsmith's approach. They remark that 360-degree feedback can help leaders in two ways. It shows them how their self-perception deviates from others' perception of their leadership, and it allows them to practice receiving feedback and turning it into a plan for development. They recommend that executives get a personal coach that will help them work on their humility. Constant feedback and coaching can help leaders improve—for better to "develop a taste for humility now than be forced to eat humble pie later" (Dame and Gedmin 2013).

4

One way a coach can help a young leader develop her humility is by helping her connect with her inner beliefs, values, and concepts. Deep in the unconscious layers of her self, each leader has core values and a worldview that has been shaped by her upbringing, experiences, and education. Imagine the core values and worldview as the most inner circle in the center of several layers of circles. The middle layers are made of talents and aptitudes, emotional intelligence (which we address in the next section), and personality preferences. The outer layers represent the visible behavior and the performance of the leader. This depiction is commonly referred to as the *leadership onion*, where outer layers of behavior are "flavored" by the inner layers of values. The inner thoughts of the leader are filtered by the middle layers and are demonstrated in the outward behaviors that her followers respond to on a daily basis (Zigarmi et al. 2005).

Most leaders don't spend enough time thinking about and reflecting on their worldview and values. Especially in healthcare, the pace of change is so rapid that leaders spend the majority of their days putting out fires, answering e-mails and voice mails, and meeting with followers and fellow executives. In this frenetic schedule, leaders don't make the effort to develop their proper center and end up adopting someone else's worldview with little intentionality. For example, concepts such as "It's business, it's not personal" and "Don't get too close to the people you lead" are often accepted by leaders as their dominant worldviews without much reflection (Hoekstra, Bell, and Peterson 2008).

The majority of leadership development and training programs tend to focus on the outer layers of behaviors without much time devoted to the inner layers of values. That narrowness is why it's important for coaches to work with leaders to intentionally examine their values. Let's take the example of Kevin, an intelligent, hard-charging, high-potential young leader working in a hospital. As an administrative resident, Kevin built an impressive resume, with several successful projects to his name. Speaking up in meetings, delivering high-quality presentations, and championing a couple of important initiatives, he caught the attention of the senior leadership team. In a few months, he was promoted to the position of assistant administrator and given significant responsibilities and several departments to manage. With a handful of directors reporting to him, his role expanded to include more growth and development of others and fewer hands-on projects.

But some of his departments were suffering from internal dysfunctionalities and conflicts that led to high unrest and turnover. To compensate, Kevin started to micromanage his direct reports and interfere with their small and big decisions. He also began to mistreat his secretary and throw tantrums every time things didn't go his way. Within six months, he was staying in his office until 9 pm or 10 pm, working harder and harder just to keep his head above the water. His bosses recognized that he was struggling and decided to send him to time management sessions and delegation training seminars, which had little impact on his ability to lead his departments effectively.

What Kevin really needs is an executive coach. Expert coaching can help him peel his leadership onion and connect with his values and worldview. In the first few sessions, the coach will work with Kevin to understand that his behaviors are mainly the result of a self-centered worldview based on the need to win at all costs and the premise that everyone should do what he wants them to do. Through some introspection, Kevin can realize that he has absorbed that worldview from others without any careful consideration. Then, the coach will start asking Kevin some deeper questions such as, "Why are you here?", "What is the purpose of your leadership in the lives that you lead?", "What contributions do you want to make?", and "What legacy do you want to leave in the world?" (Hoekstra, Bell, and Peterson 2008). As he considers these questions, Kevin will start to realize that his preferred worldview is, in fact, other-centered, and he may intentionally adopt humility, compassion, kindness, and generosity as his primary values. Per his coach's request, he'll start writing down his thoughts and reflections in a leadership journal, and he'll develop a personal mission statement. This change in the inner layers will soon be reflected in his behaviors. Instead of yelling at, micromanaging, and controlling his followers, he'll start to thank, support, and develop them. With the help of his coach, he'll embrace humility in his leadership not by focusing his efforts on changing his behavior but by deliberately reflecting on his values and worldview.

5

It's one of the most popular seminars in the history of the American College of Healthcare Executives (ACHE). Every year, at the annual Congress on Healthcare Leadership in Chicago, and at numerous other cluster meetings around the country, hundreds of healthcare leaders of all ages and levels pack the room—and even the halls—to listen to "The Courage to Lead," a seminar presented by Jody Rogers, a professor and colleague of mine at Trinity University, and George Masi, the CEO of the Harris Health System in Houston. The seminar helps leaders develop by becoming quiet but strong.

Jody is a retired lieutenant colonel from the Army Medical Service Corps who has taught leadership to executives and graduate students for the last 20 years. At Trinity, for example, he created a course that focuses on the professional development of young healthcare administration students. He locks the door to the classroom at 8 am every class session to teach students the importance of punctuality. He requires them to dress in suits for class and encourages them to think of themselves as administrators, not as students. Course topics include creating a professional presence, conducting meetings, communication skills and public speaking, social introductions, and even table etiquette—with a formal three-course dinner. His goal is to help the students enhance their leadership presence and command more respect when placed in leadership roles in their residencies and beyond.

"Can humility be taught and trained to young healthcare administrators, just like professional presence?" I asked Jody as we sat down in my office in San Antonio. "Yes, it can," he remarked in his usual serious, clear, military style. "It is about emotional intelligence and self-awareness and knowing how you respond to others and how they respond to you. Empathetic leaders know when to hug and when to give a kick in the back. They push hard but they are there when the followers need them. Yes, I believe that you can go from toxic to humble leadership, but you need self-awareness" (Rogers 2014). Jody argues that leaders who have high emotional intelligence are aware of how they treat others and how others treat them, and therefore are more likely to accurately gauge how humble they are and whether they need to make changes. A recent article on humility in management agrees with this view and states that "the humble person is aware of her status, knowledge, capabilities, strengths and weaknesses, her mistakes and limitations" (Argandona 2015, 64).

To get a better handle on the connection between emotional intelligence, self-awareness, and humility, let's go back to the origins of emotional intelligence (also called emotional quotient or EQ). In 1990, Peter Salovey from Yale University and John Mayer from the University of New Hampshire published an article in the journal *Imagination, Cognition, and Personality* titled "Emotional Intelligence." Drawing from psychological research on social intelligence, they define emotional intelligence as "the ability to monitor one's own and others' feelings and emotions, to discriminate among them, and to use this information to guide one's own thinking and actions" (Salovey and Mayer 1990, 190).

The article didn't get much attention when it was published. But soon after, while researching a story for the *New York Times*, science reporter Daniel Goleman came across it and was captivated by the notion of emotional intelligence. He spent the next five years synthesizing scientific findings and reviewing old and new theories while trying to understand how the brain regulates emotions. In 1995, Goleman published *Emotional Intelligence*, the groundbreaking book that redefined what intelligence is. He maintains that self-awareness is the keystone of emotional intelligence. Individuals who are able to monitor their feelings from moment to moment, he reasons, have better psychological insight and self-understanding, have greater certainty about their emotions, and are better able to make important decisions in their lives. Emotionally intelligent individuals aren't just aware of their own emotions but are also especially attuned to emotions in others. Building on self-awareness, Goleman emphasizes the importance of empathy as a fundamental ability (Goleman 1995).

Since the publication of Goleman's book, emotional intelligence has gone through several iterations and rounds of changes. One of the most widely accepted definitions of the concept today is "a set of emotional and social skills that influence the way we perceive and express ourselves, develop and maintain social relationships, cope with challenges, and use emotional information in an effective and meaningful way" (MHS Assessments 2017). Coaches can measure, assess, and predict executives' emotional intelligence using the Emotional Quotient Inventory (EQ-i 2.0) assessment. In this assessment, emotional intelligence is composed of five main scales: *self-perception*, *self-expression*, *interpersonal*, *decision making*, and *stress management* (see exhibit 8.1).

Self-perception consists partly of self-regard, which refers to respecting oneself while understanding and accepting one's strengths and weaknesses. It also consists of emotional self-awareness, which includes the ability to differentiate between subtleties in one's own emotions and the impact they have on one's own thoughts and actions as well as those of others. Self-expression is emotional expression (openly expressing one's feelings verbally and nonverbally) and assertiveness (communicating feelings, beliefs, and thoughts in an open way and defending personal rights and values in a nonoffensive, nondestructive manner). Interpersonal comprises interpersonal relationships, which refer to the skill of developing and maintaining mutually satisfying relationships that are characterized by trust and compassion. It also includes empathy, which is recognizing, understanding, and appreciating how other people feel. Decision making includes problem solving (understanding how emotions affect decisions), reality testing (remaining objective when making decisions), and impulse control (avoiding rash decisions and behaviors). Finally, stress management consists of flexibility (adapting to unfamiliar situations), stress tolerance (coping with stressful situations in a positive manner), and optimism (having hope despite occasional setbacks). Average scores for working professionals on these subscales typically range between 90 and 110, with 100 being the median. An extremely low score indicates a lack of a specific ability, which needs to be amplified, while an extremely high score indicates that the individual overuses an ability, which needs to be decreased.

Let's try to make sense of all of this with an example. Kate, a promising healthcare executive, has been identified by her superiors as a bit arrogant and insensitive to others' feelings. Her organization

Exhibit 8.1: Emotional Intelligence Scales and Subscales

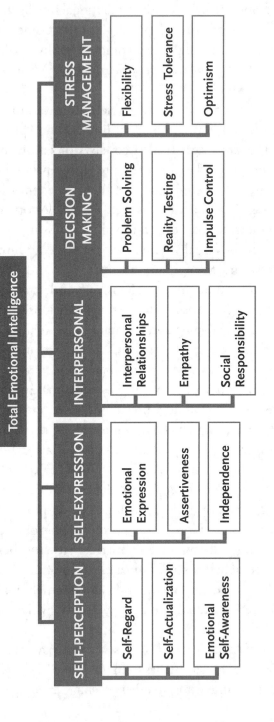

Source: Adapted from Stein and Book (2011).

can bring in an executive coach, who will administer a 360-degree evaluation for input from Kate's boss, colleagues, and subordinates, asking specifically about traits such as humility and compassion. If the feedback confirms her superiors' original impression, the coach will share it with the young executive. When she admits to her shortcomings and agrees to work on them, the coach will give her an emotional intelligence test, with a special focus on the scores received for self-regard, emotional self-awareness, assertiveness, interpersonal relationships, and empathy. An individual lacking in humility such as Kate would likely receive extremely high scores (greater than 110) on self-regard and assertiveness and extremely low scores (less than 90) on interpersonal relations and empathy. Working on the young executive's self-awareness, a customized action plan can be formulated with her coach to include specific behavioral changes and developmental goals.

For example, to address unhealthily high scores on self-regard, the coach will encourage Kate to record her reaction to any mistakes that she makes over the next few weeks. If she finds herself blaming others or blaming the system for a mistake, this tendency would indicate that she needs to start openly admitting her points of weakness. Rather than placing blame, the coach will encourage her to use mistakes as opportunities to accept her weaknesses and put in place strategies to manage them, rather than pretending they don't exist. Moreover, to deal with low scores on empathy, the coach may ask her to prepare, prior to her next staff meeting, a list of all attendees and what needs and expectations each brings to the meeting. He may ask her to try to predict how they'll act during the meeting and to anticipate what issues she needs to be sensitive to. She is also asked to generate a number of questions to further understand her colleagues' needs during the meeting.

In order to better relate with her colleagues on a personal level, the coach will encourage Kate to take the time to connect with them on topics outside of their field of work (e.g., families, children, pets, sports, current events). When the next situation that calls for empathy presents itself, she can draw on this background information to show her sensitivity to their needs (e.g., "You must be really feeling stressed with taking care of your mom, and I know your husband is traveling for work. How can I help?"). Once this action plan is in place, the coach will hold Kate accountable for the behavioral changes and evaluate her progress toward greater humility.

6

Aaron Bujnowski has three criteria for people who want to work on his team: high EQ, high IQ, and low ego. "I need them to have strong social skills, be wickedly smart, and be humble," says the senior vice president (SVP) of strategy and planning at Texas Health Resources, a network of 24 hospitals and health facilities in the North Texas region. Soft-spoken, highly intelligent, and extremely kind, Aaron is the embodiment of the Level 5 leader. His personal mission statement is to "seek to help others find meaning and direction in their lives," whereas his team's mission is to "help the organization make better decisions." He explains that both statements are outward focused, because he believes that his work and his team aren't about him but about what he can do for others and for the organization. It's what he calls *humility in action* (Bujnowski 2016):

> Humility in action, from a religious perspective, is called meekness. But I don't view it as being weak; rather, it is fierce boldness with staunch humility. For example, if you are in a meeting and someone attacks you personally, meekness is retaining self-control and not replying with a snarky comment. That takes emotional intelligence. And then you use your cognitive intelligence to come back with a thoughtful rebuttal that is focused on the issue. When you have a low ego, it is a smaller target so it is not easily

bruised. You absorb the negative energy and don't take it personally, and then you can be more thoughtful in your response. (Bujnowski 2016)

Despite the due diligence he uses when hiring new team members, he admits that he isn't always successful in hiring humble applicants. So how does he go about working with them to become more humble? "I believe in multiple pressure points," he says. One of those pressure points is modeling the behavior that you want others to repeat. "If you behave like a humble leader, others will tend to emulate you" (Bujnowski 2016). Another way is to create a culture where people correct their own behavior or correct each other. In this kind of culture, a secretary can tell the SVP that he's acting like a jerk and suffer no retaliation. On Aaron's team, that culture is based on the old cowboy saying, "Everybody ropes and everybody rides." "No one says 'I am the SVP, I don't do Excel sheets or I don't erase the board.' Whether you're the SVP or secretary, who can do the job the fastest and the best? For us, the best idea wins. It doesn't matter who comes up with it, whether it is an executive or an intern. If you have data and research behind your idea, your idea will be listened to" (Bujnowski 2016).

Another pressure point that Aaron uses to cultivate humility in his team is constant coaching and immediate feedback. For example, if he hears someone making a negative comment about another team member, he confronts her kindly and says, "When you said X, this had a negative effect on the team. Don't say X, say Y!" Or if he catches a team member acting with arrogance during a meeting, he pulls him aside after the meeting and says, "Hey man, you're way too smart to act like this. When you did that, this is how people saw you. Is this the kind of reputation you want to have? If you keep doing this you won't last long here, and I want you to be successful!" (Bujnowski 2016). Through all these tactics, Aaron believes that people can become more humble—or they eventually have to leave the organization.

The idea of modeling behavior as a way to spread humility and compassion in the organization is one that CEO Marc Strode, whom we met in chapter 7, applies on a daily basis. Every morning at 10 am, 36 directors and executives gather in the lobby of Methodist Stone Oak Hospital (MSOH) for what Marc calls the roll call. Each executive and director in this suburban San Antonio facility is assigned five patients to round on every day. Once they receive their assignments, they rush to the floors, check with the nursing units on each patient's condition, and proceed to talk to the patients. They ask the patients about their stay, how responsive the nurses are, and whether their pain is well managed. They inquire about the food, the call buttons and television channels, and whether they can make their experience better. Then they thank the patients for choosing MSOH as their preferred hospital. After finishing their rounds, the executives and directors follow up with the unit's providers on the issues that the patients may have raised. They take the time to share positive feedback with the team in order to reinforce positive behaviors.

Marc started roll call in August of 2015. The executives and directors have rounded on patients *every single day* since then. "When I first introduced the idea to the team, they looked at me like I was crazy," Marc recounts. They came up with every excuse to not do it. "Especially our finance and IT [information technology] people, they were terrified." Some of them said that they had important meetings they couldn't miss. "Reschedule them!" Marc replied. Others argued they had to attend systemwide conference calls. "I will take care of all the system stuff—don't worry about it. You just show up at 10 am every morning and round," said Marc, having already gotten the approval from his boss, the system CEO (Strode 2016). He wanted to make sure that all of the patients in his hospital on any given day were visited by one member of the leadership team at least once every 24 hours. Someone on his team had told him that if you do something for 21 days, it becomes a habit. So he circled that specific day on his calendar and kept pushing his team until the rounding became a habit, and the leaders finally started enjoying it.

One Friday last fall, Marc invited me to make the rounds with him. He looked very relaxed that morning in his jeans and cowboy boots. When we reached the surgical unit that he was assigned to that day, he rolled up his sleeves and sat down to talk to the nurse in charge of his five patients. It looked like the most natural thing in the world—the nurse explaining clinical terms, and the CEO listening intently and scribbling notes. One of our patients was an elderly woman who was there for her fifth surgery. When we entered the room, Marc humbly introduced himself as the CEO of the hospital. The woman's eyes lit up in excitement. He then pulled a chair up to her bed. When she told him about her repeated health problems, he held her hand and listened attentively. When she told him about the delays in her discharge, he promised to follow up with her physician. Then he gave her his personal card and wrote his cell phone number on it, asking her to call him if she needed anything. He repeated the procedure with the other four patients. It was humility and compassion in action.

"Why have you insisted so much on rounding on patients every day?" I asked Marc as we sat down in his Texas-themed office after. "Rounding is just a tactic; it's not effective without having relationships with the staff. When the nurses and other staff see me do that day in and day out, they say, 'This is the place I want to be,'" he explained (Strode 2016). Other CEOs from other hospitals have told him that this approach of rounding every day for two hours, while he has a hospital to run and a $150 million building project next door, wouldn't be sustainable.

> That was even more of a challenge to us because I know it works. It is a fundamental approach that defines our culture. It is not just about feeling good—it impacts our results. As people buy into rounding, it leads to lower turnover, so we don't have to spend time on hiring and training.

Our variability in processes goes down, which makes us safer. Our labor costs go down as well and our loyalty goes up. This is my argument. Having perfected this for over a year now and seeing the positive impact the exercise has not only on our patients but our nurses, our housekeepers, our physicians, I couldn't imagine leading a hospital and not doing this consistently on a daily basis. (Strode 2016)

Marc had learned about the importance of rounding from his first preceptor during his administrative residency at Methodist Hospital in San Antonio. "I have rounded since my first day on January 5, 1998. Nearly 20 years later, I am still rounding. Not once has it gone old for me," he adds, brimming with pride (Strode 2016). Just as Marc does, young careerists can learn about ways to practice humility and compassion from their bosses and mentors.

8

As an up-and-coming leader, you may be starting to wonder: How do I start working on being more humble and treating my subordinates with compassion and kindness? At the risk of providing prescriptive actions and specific-step models (which I promised you I wouldn't do), in this section, I'll share a few ideas that can help you get started. Some of these ideas will make more sense to you than others, so I encourage you to pick and choose what fits your personality, needs, position, and organization.

Any improvement in humility and compassion has to start with some work on your own. You can develop yourself as a compassionate leader by creating mental habits. (Warning—things are about to get New Agey!) The idea behind mental habits is that the more you think about something, the stronger the required neural pathways become. When the pathways improve, it becomes easier for you to have that thought—it becomes a mental habit, a frequent and effortless thought. For example, to work on becoming more compassionate, you can train your brain to think about goodness. This effort would include three mental habits:

1. Thinking about and seeing goodness in yourself and others
2. Giving goodness to all
3. Believing that you can multiply goodness (Tan 2010, 199)

As you might recall from a previous chapter, compassion includes three components: the affective portion ("I feel for you"), the cognitive portion ("I understand you"), and the motivational portion ("I want to help you"). The first habit of thinking about and seeing goodness in yourself and others can help you strengthen the affective and cognitive aspects of compassion. This habit starts with meditating about how good you are as a person, and how good other people are. When you train yourself to think about this frequently, you begin perceiving goodness in everyone, and you instinctively want to understand and feel for them. This process applies, for example, in difficult situations, such as a meeting in which a colleague is behaving poorly. Instead of simply dismissing his actions with a "that's just the way he is," thinking about goodness will make you want to understand that colleague, because you know there's at least a hint of goodness in him. For example, you may ask if his family is doing well or whether his boss is putting a lot of pressure on him. As you practice this mental habit more and more, eventually people will see you as someone they can trust, because you understand them and care about them (Tan 2010).

The second habit, giving goodness to others, can help you strengthen the motivational component of compassion. When you start constantly thinking about delivering goodness to the world, you become a person who always wants to help others. As you make it a habit to coach your subordinates or help your colleagues with their projects, people will know that your heart is in the right place, and you become a leader that people respect and admire.

The last habit, becoming confident in your ability to multiply goodness, can help your self-confidence. When you constantly think about and reflect on your transformative power, you become comfortable with the idea of becoming an agent of goodness. You start thinking, "Yes, I can benefit people." The more people you help, the more you'll be seen as an inspirational leader (Tan 2010).

To develop those mental habits, some self-taught, simple meditation techniques can go a long way. For example, visualization is a powerful mental tool that's easy to learn. The idea behind visualization is that our brains are forced to devote a substantial amount of resources to processing a visual image—so when we create a mental image, we push our brain's computational resources, which makes it stick. For example, to develop the three mental habits needed for compassion, you can visualize your goodness as a white light. In your meditation, focus on your breathing and imagine that you're breathing in your own goodness. Then visualize yourself multiplying that goodness by ten in your heart. After that, when you exhale, visualize that you're giving all that goodness to the world.

For those who are more serious about their meditation and about developing compassion, several rigorous training programs are available. Some of those started with the work of Dr. Tania Singer at the Institute for Human Cognitive and Brain Sciences in Leipzig, Germany. A few years ago, Singer and her team began to study the plasticity of the social brain, a line of research that includes whether socioaffective skills, such as compassion and empathy, can be trained and whether that mental training can influence psychological and physical well-being and social behavior. Out of this research came several mental training programs for the improvement of compassion and empathy (Singer and Bolz 2013). For example, mindful self-compassion training is an eight-week program of self-transformation in which participants practice breathing, meditation, and self-compassionate letter writing, among other activities. Drawing from Tibetan Buddhist traditions, cognitively based compassion training is a system of "mind training" that focuses on cognitive and analytical meditation techniques to help participants reframe their relationships with others.

But sitting on a mat and breathing in and out can only take you so far. You obviously have to practice your compassion with others. The first step in that process is to be in the present—coming into the moment of interacting without any prejudice or desires based on past experience or former relations. "Compassion without history and desire brings equanimity—a more even mind or temperament, more often referred to as balancing our heart with our head," notes Geoff Aigner, the Australian leadership expert we discussed in chapters 3 and 4 (Aigner 2010, 62). A practical way to develop this composure and mental calmness is to listen. As a leader, really listening to your employees and understanding their concerns is much more effective than constantly offering suggestions and trying to fix problems. When leaders listen, they truly focus while seeking to understand, which creates energy and spurs their followers' imagination. Robert Greenleaf, creator of the notion of servant leadership, remarked long ago that servant leaders' first reaction to any problem is to listen (Greenleaf 1970).

In his excellent book *The Coaching Habit*, Canadian coach Michael Bungay Stanier echoes this view and argues that leaders should listen more, commit to asking more questions, and give less advice. In that sense, the leader behaves more like a coach who mentors employees instead of doing their work for them. Stanier emphasizes the importance of leaders focusing on *coaching for development*, which develops the person trying to solve the problem ("focus on the firefighter") more than *coaching for performance*, which can help solve everyday managerial problems ("focus on putting out fires"). Some of the questions that he recommends leaders frequently ask their employees are "What's on your mind?", "What is the real challenge here for you?", "What do you want?", and finally, "How can I help?" (Stanier 2016).

Similarly, coaches Erik Hoekstra, Antony Bell, and Scott Peterson emphasize the importance of listening and asking questions when they work with leaders seeking to increase their humility. In their coaching sessions, they ask leaders to self-report two pairs of statistics. One is the amount of time they spend during meetings and in sessions with followers making statements and the amount of time they spend asking questions. The second is the percentage of the time they spend during a typical day speaking and listening. For leaders who are low on humility, the ratio of statements to questions is about 10:1, whereas the percentage of listening time is typically less than 20 percent. The coaches note that unless these numbers change, leaders cannot develop true humility (Hoekstra, Bell, and Peterson 2008).

Another way to show compassion toward followers is to trust them. When you trust your employees, you allow them to make their own decisions and provide support for them to carry out their plans. If you have highly capable and intelligent employees, you'll be better off trusting them to decide than telling them what they should do. However, trust cannot be blind. "Our trust needs to be tempered with setting boundaries. After all, we want to be around to fight another day. Compassion is not some endless, bleeding, open heart" comments Aigner (2010, 64). Compassion-ate leaders trust others, which requires them to realize that they're not always in control. As part of that process, they start replacing control with creativity. When you constantly feel that you have to be in control of what is happening and how people are reacting, you run the risk of becoming rigid and not having the necessary creative intelligence to be available for your employees in a useful way (Aigner 2010).

Compassion, which is based on listening, trust, and creativity, can be applied in small daily interactions such as checking on employees and managing their performance. It can also be very useful in major organizational changes such as layoffs, in which the leader has no control over events. "Sometimes we don't have anything to give to people but our ears and our presence. We are all that is providing direction, protection, order, and care," Aigner suggests (2010, 65). In difficult situations marred by uncertainty and anxiety, a compas-sionate leader makes herself available to listen to fears and concerns, even if she can't necessarily solve the problems.

9

The average millennial spends one hour per week taking selfies. On average, if she keeps taking selfies at that rate, she'll have taken 26,000 over her lifetime. Each selfie consumes seven minutes of her precious time, spent on taking the picture, editing it, realizing that her hair looks bad, retaking it, editing the new one, deciding on a caption and emoji, and finally posting it on social media (Papisova 2016). Parenting expert Dr. Michele Borba calls this self-absorbed craze the *selfie epidemic*, which she describes as an obsession with self-promotion, personal branding, and self-interest with no regard for others' feelings, needs, and concerns (Borba 2016b). In her recent book *UnSelfie*, Borba argues that the best way to fight the "I, me, and mine" obsession is with empathy, which is the foundation of humanity.

While preparing for her book, she travelled around the world to places such as Phnom Penh, Dachau, Auschwitz, and Rwanda to see inhumanity and empathy in action. These powerful visits made her realize that a strong sense of empathy is necessary for young people to attain health, happiness, and career success. She also realized that empathy isn't an innate trait—rather, like the idea that two plus two equals four, it's one that can be taught to schoolchildren. "When children can grasp another's perspective, they are more likely to be empathetic, anticipate the other's behavior or thinking, handle conflicts peacefully, be less judgmental, value differences, speak up for those who are victimized, and act in ways that are more helpful, comforting, and supportive of others," she notes (Borba 2016a). Kids who understand others' points of view acquire the *unselfie empathy advantage*: They're better adjusted, have healthier relations with their peers, and are better prepared for the demands of leadership in the workplace.

To obtain the empathy advantage, Borba recommends that children and young adults practice some teachable habits, such as emotional literacy, moral identity, perspective taking, moral imagination, self-regulation, kindness, collaboration, moral courage, and compassionate leadership abilities. For example, teaching children to recognize and understand the feelings and needs of others in their body language, tone of voice, or facial expressions can help them develop emotional literacy. Helping them develop ethical codes and caring mind-sets will make them more likely to adopt caring values that define their moral identities. Forcing them to stretch their perspectives allows them to step into others' shoes to understand feelings, thoughts, and views. These habits can, in turn, enable children to practice kindness by training them in prosocial behaviors that increase their concern about the welfare and feelings of others and enhance the likelihood that they'll step in to help, support, or comfort others. Eventually, children will be able to cultivate their altruistic leadership abilities to be motivated to make a difference for those who work with them and for them (Borba 2017).

Spearheaded by Borba's efforts, many of these habits are being taught to children in schools all over the country. She tells the story of one school where the principal was helping his students practice perspective taking:

> I was visiting a Kansas school when I happened upon two boys engaged in serious conversation with their principal. The eleven-year-olds were in trouble (again) for another "heated" debate over their shared locker and had escalated to a physical confrontation. Each accused the other of "messing with my stuff," but the principal was using a different discipline ploy. She handed each a "Think Sheet," which required the boys to answer from the other's perspective. Questions on her "Think Sheet" included:
> "What happened?"
> "What would the other person say happened?"
> "How do you feel about what happened?"
> "How do you think the other person feels or needs?"
> "What would you like to tell the other person?"

"What is the best way to solve this problem so both of you are satisfied?"

Listening to their reactions was priceless:

"I'm not him, so how do I know how he feels?"

"This is too hard," said the other. "I can't figure out what he wants."

And that was their problem: neither thought about how the other felt because each was seeing only "their side."

The principal's perspective-taking strategy was a brilliant way to help the boys figure out the feelings, thoughts, and needs of someone beside themselves. And in today's selfie-absorbed world, that strategy is crucial (Borba 2017).

Examples of programs implemented in other schools include making students literally put themselves in other people's shoes by trying on an oversized shoe, rewriting stories using the first person, holding 24-hour voluntary fasts, and asking students to move around the classroom with a blindfold on. While I'm not suggesting that healthcare administration programs should necessarily adopt these practices, Borba's approach is a reminder that positive leadership traits such as empathy can be learned through intentional practices.

10

In this chapter, I've described several practices and techniques that can help you cultivate humility, compassion, and empathy. If these have sounded like huge commitments of time and energy, here's an easy way for you to begin looking like a humble leader: Start making fun of yourself! In a study conducted by the Bell Leadership Institute in Chapel Hill, North Carolina, when employees were asked to describe the strengths of their senior colleagues, "sense of humor" was mentioned twice as much as any other trait. The research found that the most effective leaders used humor to spark their followers' enthusiasm, deliver honest messages in an easy-to-accept way, put their employees at ease, and see the light side in difficult situations (Bell Leadership Institute 2012). Similarly, research by the executive recruitment firm Robert Half International concluded that 90 percent of employed professionals believe that humor is important for career advancement, with 84 percent of them agreeing that people with a good sense of humor are better employees (Wilkie 2013).

The most effective type of humor for leaders is self-deprecating humor. Leaders who use this kind of humor are rated as being more attentive and sensitive to their followers' individual needs and skills, an important aspect of humility (Hoption, Barling, and Turner 2013). Stan Hupfeld, the generous healthcare leader from Oklahoma whom we met in chapter 5, argues that "the ultimate act of humility is to not take yourself too seriously in a very serious business; self-deprecating humor is a way to endear the leader to his/her staff" (Hupfeld 2016). This opinion is in line with evidence from other studies showing that leaders who use self-deprecating humor are willing to make themselves potentially vulnerable by identifying their weaknesses to others (Westwood 2004). In that sense, humor can help the leader be seen as closer to or at the same level as his followers (Kets de Vries 1990; Martin et al. 2003). Leaders who can laugh at themselves are perceived as more likable than those who take themselves too seriously, which can benefit their relationships with their followers (Ziv 1984). Moreover, self-deprecating humor is positively correlated with the ability to persuade others, which is important for leaders trying to get their followers to implement major initiatives (Lyttle 2001).

President Dwight D. Eisenhower is reputed to have once said: "A sense of humor is part of the art of leadership, of getting along with people, of getting things done." So take Ike's advice, loosen up a bit, and use self-deprecating humor to your advantage. For instance, next time you're introducing a new team member to your group, you can end your little speech by saying something like, "I'm glad Mary has taken this job despite knowing all about me!" Become more comfortable with the idea of laughing at yourself and allowing others to join you. You may be surprised how this will help you come across as more vulnerable, more likable, and more humble, and how it will boost your leadership effectiveness.

But before I let you go, I need to warn you that self-deprecating humor isn't the same thing as humblebragging. *Humblebragging* is a term coined by the late comedian, actor, and writer Harris Wittels to refer to a specific type of a brag that masks the boasting part of a statement in a falsely humble guise. The false humility allows the person to boast about his achievement without guilt (Wittels 2012). While the statement is typically self-deprecating in nature, its actual purpose is to draw attention to something of which one is proud. For example, Matt recently was nominated as one of the "best leaders under 40" by his local ACHE chapter. To promote his achievement among his friends while appearing humble, he updated his Facebook status: "Just got nominated for an ACHE award. Have to give a fancy acceptance speech—SCARY!!!" Don't be like Matt. Humblebragging is annoying (Alford 2012), and as a recent study has shown, it's not effective as a self-promotional strategy (Sezer, Gino, and Norton 2015). Be humble and let your actions speak for themselves.

11

By now I hope that you're starting to realize that cultivating humility and compassion is hard work but is also worth all the time and energy. Benjamin Franklin spent a lot of effort on stifling his pride and improving his humility. Even if he wasn't completely successful, at least he managed the appearance of success, which helped him win more arguments and support.

> The modest way in which I proposed my opinions procured them a readier reception and less contradiction; I had less mortification when I was found to be in the wrong, and I more easily prevailed with others to give up their mistakes and join with me when I happened to be in the right. . . . And to this habit (after my character of integrity) I think

it principally owing that I had early so much weight with my fellow-citizens when I proposed new institutions, or alterations in the old, and so much influence in public councils when I became a member. (Franklin 2017, 97)

Franklin's arduous attempts to conquer his ego, despite their limited success, allowed him to be better received by others, an important factor in becoming one of the most influential leaders in the history of our country. His example is an important reminder for you as a young leader to start your journey toward the leadership intangibles of humility, compassion, kindness, and generosity. Before too long, people will start seeing you as a humbitious leader who drives high performance in your organization.

REFERENCES

Aigner, G. 2010. *Leadership Beyond Good Intentions: What It Takes to Really Make a Difference.* Crows Nest, Australia: Allen & Unwin.

Alford, H. 2012. "If I Do Humblebrag So Myself." *New York Times.* Published November 30. www.nytimes.com/2012/12/02/fashion/bah-humblebrag-the-unfortunate-rise-of-false-humility.html.

Argandona, A. 2015. "Humility in Management." *Journal of Business Ethics* 132 (1): 63–71.

Arruda, W. 2014. "Why You Need to Hire a Coach in 2015." *Forbes.* Published December 9. www.forbes.com/sites/williamarruda/2014/12/09/why-you-need-to-hire-a-coach-in-2015/#3eb1ec624de3.

Barboza, D. 1995. "Darwin E. Smith, 69, Executive Who Remade a Paper Company." *New York Times.* Published December 28. www.nytimes.com/1995/12/28/us/darwin-e-smith-69-executive-who-remade-a-paper-company.html.

Bell Leadership Institute. 2012. "Bell Leadership Study Finds Humor Gives Leaders the Edge." Published March. www.bell leadership.com/humor-gives-leaders-edge/.

Bobb, D. J. 2013. *Humility: An Unlikely Biography of America's Greatest Virtue*. Nashville, TN: Nelson Books.

Borba, M. 2017. "7 Ways to Teach Perspective Taking and Stretch Students' Empathy Muscles." MicheleBorba.com. Accessed March 20. http://micheleborba.com/8-ways-to-teach-perspective-taking-and-stretch-students-empathy-muscles/.

———. 2016a. "Seven Ways to Raise Caring Kids." *Medium*. Published July 15. https://medium.com/galleys/7-ways-to -raise-caring-kids-3badbb2fac86.

———. 2016b. *UnSelfie: Why Empathetic Kids Succeed in Our All-About-Me World*. New York: Touchstone.

Bujnowski, A. 2016. Phone interview. September 19.

Campbell, J. 1999. *Recovering Benjamin Franklin: An Exploration of a Life of Science and Service*. Chicago: Open Court.

Collins, J. 2001. *Good to Great: Why Some Companies Make the Leap . . . and Others Don't*. New York: Harper Business.

Dame, J., and J. Gedmin. 2013. "Six Principles for Developing Humility as a Leader." *Harvard Business Review*. Published September 9. https://hbr.org/2013/09/six-principles-for-developing.

Eliot, C. W. (ed.). 2010. *Benjamin Franklin, John Woolman, and William Penn*. The Five Foot Shelf of Classics. Vol. 1. New York: Cosimo Classics.

Franklin, B. 2017. *The Autobiography of Benjamin Franklin: The Complete Illustrated History*. Minneapolis: Voyageur Press.

Goldsmith, M. 2017. "Self Assessment: Leadership Excellence." MarshallGoldsmith.com. Accessed April 6. www.marshallgold smith.com/articles/self-assessment/.

————. 2007. *What Got You Here Won't Get You There: How Successful People Become Even More Successful.* New York: Hyperion Books.

Goleman, D. 1995. *Emotional Intelligence.* New York: Bantam Books.

Greenleaf, R. K. 1970. *The Servant as Leader.* Indianapolis: The Robert K. Greenleaf Center for Servant Leadership.

Hoekstra, E., A. Bell, and S. R. Peterson. 2008. "Humility in Leadership: Abandoning the Pursuit of Unattainable Perfection." In *Executive Ethics: Ethical Dilemmas and Challenges for the C-Suite,* edited by S. A. Quatro and R. R. Sims, 79–95. Greenwich, CT: Information Age Publishing.

Hoption, C., J. Barling, and N. Turner. 2013. "'It's Not You, It's Me': Transformational Leadership and Self-deprecating Humor." *Leadership and Organization Development Journal* 34 (1): 4–19.

Hupfeld, S. 2016. E-mail correspondence with the author. December 21.

Kets de Vries, M. F. R. 1990. "The Organizational Fool: Balancing a Leader's Hubris." *Human Relations* 43 (8): 751–70.

Lyttle, J. 2001. "The Effectiveness of Humor in Persuasion: The Case of Business Ethics Training." *Journal of General Psychology* 128 (2): 206–16.

Martin, R. A., P. Puhlik-Doris, G. Larsen, J. Gray, and K. Weir. 2003. "Individual Differences in Uses of Humor and Their Relation to Psychological Well-Being: Development of the Humor Styles Questionnaire." *Journal of Research in Personality* 37 (1): 48–75.

MHS Assessments. 2017. "About Emotional Intelligence." Accessed April 7. https://tap.mhs.com/AboutEmotional Intelligence.aspx.

Papisova, V. 2016. "Fun Fact: Millennials Dedicate One Hour Each Week to Selfies." *Teen Vogue*. www.teenvogue.com/story /millennials-instagram-selfies-study.

Rogers, J. 2014. Personal interview. November 6.

Salovey, P., and J. D. Mayer. 1990. "Emotional Intelligence." *Imagination, Cognition, and Personality* 9 (3): 185–211.

Sezer, O., F. Gino, and M. J. Norton. 2015. "Humblebragging: A Distinct—and Ineffective—Self-Presentation Strategy." Working Paper 15-080, Harvard Business School.

Singer, T., and M. Bolz. 2013. *Compassion: Bridging Science and Practice*. Munich: Max Planck Society.

Stanier, M. B. 2016. *The Coaching Habit: Say Less, Ask More, and Change the Way You Lead Forever*. Toronto: Box of Crayons Press.

Stein, S. J., and H. E. Book. 2011. *The EQ Edge: Emotional Intelligence and Your Success*. San Francisco: Jossey-Bass.

Strode, M. 2016. Personal interview. September 26.

Tan, C. 2010. *Search Inside Yourself: The Unexpected Path to Achieving Success, Happiness (and World Peace)*. New York: HarperOne.

Tangney, J. P. 2000. "Humility: Theoretical Perspectives, Empirical Findings and Directions for Future Research." *Journal of Social and Clinical Psychology* 19 (1): 70–82.

Westwood, R. 2004. "Comic Relief: Subversion and Catharsis in Organizational Comedic Theatre." *Organization Studies* 25 (5): 775–95.

Wilkie, D. 2013. "Inside Joke: Humor Can Help the Bottom Line." Society for Human Resource Management. Published October. www .shrm.org/resourcesandtools/hr-topics/employee-relations /pages/jokes-humor-workplace.aspx.

Wittels, H. 2012. *Humblebrag: The Art of False Modesty*. New York: Grand Central Publishing.

Worthington, E. 2007. *Humility: The Quiet Virtue*. Philadelphia: Templeton Foundation Press.

Zigarmi, D., K. Blanchard, M. O'Connor, and C. Edeburn. 2005. *The Leader Within*. Upper Saddle River, NJ: Prentice Hall.

Ziv, A. 1984. *Personality and Sense of Humor*. New York: Springer.

Research Methods

To supplement the secondary research reported in this book, I collected qualitative and quantitative data. First, I conducted in-depth interviews with 20 current and previous healthcare leaders, providers, and experts on leadership-related issues. The interviews were done in person or by phone and they lasted between 45 and 75 minutes.

With some variations, the questions asked included but were not limited to the following:

- What is your view on the importance of humility in healthcare leadership?
- What is your view on the importance of compassion in healthcare leadership?
- What is your view on the importance of kindness in healthcare leadership?
- What is your view on the importance of generosity in healthcare leadership?
- What are examples of these types of traits in leaders that you have encountered in your career?
- What are the advantages of these traits to the leader and organization?
- What are the disadvantages of these traits to the leader and organization?

- Can these traits work against the leader? Can he be taken advantage of?
- Is it harder or easier to demonstrate these traits when you are early in your career than when you are already an established leader?
- Is there a difference between generations in exhibiting these traits?
- Is there a difference between men and women in exhibiting these traits?
- Can these traits be learned and trained for?
- Have you encountered leaders who have exhibited characteristics different from these traits? For example, arrogant, self-centered, cruel, and so on?

The list of interviewees in alphabetical order is included in exhibit 1.

Exhibit 1: List of Interviewees

Interviewee	Title
Don Beeler	Chief Executive Officer (retired), CHRISTUS Santa Rosa Healthcare System, San Antonio, Texas
Aaron Bujnowski	Senior Vice President, Strategy and Planning, Texas Health Resources, Dallas, Texas
Enrique Gallegos	Chief Executive Officer, Laredo Medical Center, Laredo, Texas
Dr. Gary Greensweig	Vice President and Chief Physician Executive for Physician Integration, Dignity Health, San Francisco, California
Gordon Hawthorne	Vice Chair and Healthcare Practice Leader, Diversified Search, Philadelphia, Pennsylvania
John Hornbeak	Chief Executive Officer (retired), Methodist Healthcare System, San Antonio, Texas
Stanley Hupfeld	Chief Executive Officer (retired), INTEGRIS Health, Oklahoma City, Oklahoma

Exhibit 1: List of Interviewees *(continued)*

Interviewee	Title
Sally Hurt-Deitch	Chief Executive Officer, The Hospitals of Providence, El Paso, Texas
Rebecca Ivatury	Charge Nurse (retired), US Air Force, San Antonio, Texas; Administrative Resident (former), Methodist Healthcare, San Antonio, Texas
Amelie Karam	Millennial Specialist, Speaker, and Consultant, Nashville, Tennessee
Edward Lamb	CEO, Mount Carmel Health System, Columbus, Ohio; Chairman, American College of Healthcare Executives (former), Chicago, Illinois
Jennifer Malatek	Coach, Studer Group, Pensacola, Florida; Chief Executive Officer (former), Ernest Health, New Braunfels, Texas
Heidi Pandya	Director, Health Industries Advisory, PricewaterhouseCoopers, Dallas, Texas
Jody Rogers	Visiting Professor, Trinity University, San Antonio, Texas; Faculty Member, American College of Healthcare Executives, Chicago, Illinois
Robert Shaw	President (retired), Norton Cancer Institute, Louisville, Kentucky
Corinne Smith	Partner, Strasburger & Price, LLP, Austin, Texas; Director (former), Legal Services, Seton Healthcare Family, Austin, Texas
Hurley Smith	Senior Consultant, Stanford Health Care, Palo Alto, California
Marc Strode	Chief Executive Officer, Methodist Stone Oak Hospital, San Antonio, Texas
Phil Wentworth	Chief Executive Officer (retired), Texas Health Resources Plano, Plano, Texas
Michael Zucker	Chief Executive Officer and Cofounder, Ranger Health, Inc., San Antonio, Texas

Second, I conducted a quantitative survey of employees, supervisors or frontline managers, middle managers, and executives working in a convenience sample of nine healthcare organizations. An e-mail request was sent to an executive in the organization asking for permission to collect the data. Once that permission was granted, a link to a SurveyMonkey questionnaire was sent to the executive. The executive addressed an e-mail to the relevant employee groups in his organization asking for their participation in the questionnaire and guaranteeing anonymity. Some organizations agreed to send the questionnaire to all their employees, while others limited it to the executive suite or to all executives and middle managers. I received 577 completed surveys, for a response rate of 29 percent, which is typical in surveys involving healthcare managers and professionals. The profiles of the organizations and the number of respondents per organization are described in exhibit 2.

Exhibit 2: Organizational Profile of Survey Respondents

Organization Type	Location	Requests	Respondents	Response Rate (%)
Not-for-profit health system	Oklahoma City	230	76	33
For-profit hospital	North Texas	47	17	36
For-profit hospital	South Texas	685	115	17
For-profit hospital	San Antonio	34	22	65
Not-for-profit hospital	South Texas	4	3	75
For-profit health system	South Texas	160	45	28
For-profit hospital	San Antonio	44	18	41
Not-for-profit health system	Northwest Texas	20	7	35
Public physician group	San Antonio	760	274	36
Total		**1984**	**577**	**29**

The following tables provide a breakdown of respondents by organization type, age, gender, and position.

Exhibit 3: Respondents by Organizational Type

Organization Type	Number	Percentage
For-profit	217	37.6
Not-for-profit/public	360	62.4
Total	**577**	**100**

Exhibit 4: Respondents by Organizational Level

Organizational Level	Number	Percentage
Employee	285	49.4
Supervisor/frontline manager	57	9.9
Middle manager/ director	183	31.7
Executive	51	8.8
Total	**576**	**100**

Exhibit 5: Respondents by Gender

Gender	Number	Percentage
Female	416	72.3
Male	159	27.7
Total	**575**	**100**

Exhibit 6: Respondents by Age Group

Age Group	Number	Percentage
18–34 years	95	16.5
35–54 years	331	57.4
55–74 years	147	25.5
Total	573	100

The questionnaire consisted of, in addition to the organizational and demographic questions, four main questions:

1. Think about the leader that has had the most positive influence on your career; someone you know personally. Please indicate that leader's gender: male/female
   Choose up to 5 terms that best describe him/her.

Humble	Arrogant
Compassionate	Holds others accountable
Blames others	Kind
Empathetic	Inconsiderate
Self-focused	Accountable
Generous	Harsh
Insensitive	Passive

2. Think about the one leader that you have observed to be the most successful in terms of improving outcomes (quality, financial, etc.) in the organization and getting things done; someone you know personally (could be the same leader you chose for the previous question or someone different). Please indicate that leader's gender: male/female

Choose up to 5 terms that best describe him/her.

Humble	Arrogant
Compassionate	Holds others accountable
Blames others	Kind
Empathetic	Inconsiderate
Self-focused	Accountable
Generous	Harsh
Insensitive	Passive

3. Think about the one leader that has had a negative influence on your career; someone you know personally (could be the same leader you chose for a previous question or someone different). Please indicate that leader's gender: male/female

   Choose up to 5 terms that best describe him/her.

Humble	Arrogant
Compassionate	Holds others accountable
Blames others	Kind
Empathetic	Inconsiderate
Self-focused	Accountable
Generous	Harsh
Insensitive	Passive

4. Think about the one leader that you have observed to be the least successful in terms of improving outcomes (quality, financial, etc.) in the organization and getting things done; someone you know personally (could be the same leader you chose for a previous question or someone different). Please indicate that leader's gender: male/female

Choose up to 5 terms that best describe him/her.

Humble	Arrogant
Compassionate	Holds others accountable
Blames others	Kind
Empathetic	Inconsiderate
Self-focused	Accountable
Generous	Harsh
Insensitive	Passive

To prevent respondents from automatically choosing the same traits for every question, I used the SurveyMonkey feature that allows for the traits to be presented randomly for each question.

The following tables include all the responses to the four questions, organized by frequency of answers:

Exhibit 7: Traits of Leaders with Positive Influence (Ranked)

Traits	Number	Percentage
Accountable	343	59.4
Compassionate	297	51.5
Collaborative	290	50.3
Calm	274	47.5
Kind	259	44.9
Holds others accountable	241	41.8
Humble	219	38.0
Generous	204	35.4
Ambitious	187	32.4
Empathetic	143	24.8
Charismatic	140	24.3
Self-focused	64	11.1

Exhibit 7: Traits of Leaders with Positive Influence (Ranked) *(continued)*

Traits	Number	Percentage
Passive	25	4.3
Harsh	9	1.6
Condescending	9	1.6
Insensitive	8	1.4
Inconsiderate	6	1.0
Blames others	4	0.7
Arrogant	3	0.5
Dishonest	1	0.2

Exhibit 8: Gender of Leaders with Positive Influence

Gender	Number	Percentage
Female	314	54.7
Male	260	45.3
Total	574	100

Exhibit 9: Traits of Successful Leaders (Ranked)

Traits	Number	Percentage
Accountable	368	63.8
Collaborative	311	53.9
Holds others accountable	279	48.4
Calm	229	39.7
Compassionate	226	39.2
Ambitious	226	39.2
Kind	221	38.3

(continued)

Exhibit 9: Traits of Successful Leaders (Ranked) *(continued)*

Traits	Number	Percentage
Humble	172	29.8
Generous	166	28.8
Charismatic	159	27.6
Empathetic	99	17.2
Self-focused	84	14.6
Passive	31	5.4
Harsh	20	3.5
Arrogant	13	2.3
Condescending	13	2.3
Insensitive	12	2.1
Inconsiderate	11	1.9
Dishonest	7	1.2
Blames others	5	0.9

Exhibit 10: Gender of Successful Leaders

Gender	Number	Percentage
Female	296	51.7
Male	276	48.3
Total	**572**	**100**

Exhibit 11: Traits of Leaders with Negative Influence (Ranked)

Traits	Number	Percentage
Arrogant	301	52.2
Inconsiderate	291	50.4
Condescending	291	50.4
Blames others	289	50.1
Self-focused	269	46.6
Insensitive	267	46.3
Harsh	216	37.4
Dishonest	201	34.8
Ambitious	94	16.3
Holds others accountable	90	15.6
Passive	75	13.0
Charismatic	38	6.6
Calm	29	5.0
Accountable	24	4.2
Empathetic	18	3.1
Kind	17	2.9
Generous	14	2.4
Collaborative	14	2.4
Humble	11	1.9
Compassionate	9	1.6

Exhibit 12: Gender of Leaders with Negative Influence

Gender	Number	Percentage
Female	296	51.5
Male	278	49.5
Total	574	100

Exhibit 13: Traits of Unsuccessful Leaders (Ranked)

Traits	Number	Percentage
Blames others	295	51.1
Self-focused	255	44.2
Arrogant	243	42.1
Insensitive	229	39.7
Condescending	205	35.5
Dishonest	181	31.4
Harsh	170	29.5
Passive	157	27.2
Holds others accountable	72	12.5
Ambitious	70	12.1
Calm	68	11.8
Kind	63	10.9
Charismatic	37	6.4
Generous	34	5.9
Empathetic	32	5.5
Compassionate	31	5.4
Humble	28	4.9
Accountable	22	3.8
Collaborative	21	3.6
Inconsiderate	24	3.2

Exhibit 14: Gender of Unsuccessful Leaders

Gender	Number	Percentage
Female	277	48.9
Male	289	51.1
Total	566	100

To gain a better understanding of the differences in perceptions between men and women, I conducted the following analyses by gender.

Exhibit 15: Traits of Leaders with Positive Influence (by Respondent Gender)

Traits	Female Respondents	Male Respondents
Accountable	248 (60%)	93 (59%)
Ambitious	132 (32%)	55 (35%)
Arrogant	3 (1%)	0 (0%)
Blames others	4 (1%)	0 (0%)
Calm	196 (47%)	77 (48%)
Charismatic	91 (22%)	49 (31%)
Collaborative	206 (50%)	83 (52%)
Compassionate	225 (54%)	70 (44%)
Condescending	4 (1%)	5 (3%)
Dishonest	1 (0%)	0 (0%)
Empathetic	114 (27%)	27 (17%)
Generous	147 (35%)	57 (36%)
Harsh	9 (2%)	0 (0%)
Holds others accountable	172 (41%)	68 (43%)
Humble	149 (36%)	70 (44%)
Inconsiderate	5 (1%)	1 (1%)
Insensitive	7 (2%)	1 (1%)
Kind	200 (48%)	58 (37%)
Passive	16 (4%)	9 (6%)
Self-focused	45 (11%)	19 (12%)
Total	416 (100%)	159 (100%)

Exhibit 16: Top Five Traits of Leaders with Positive Influence (by Respondent Gender)

Female Respondents	Male Respondents
Accountable (60%)	Accountable (59%)
Compassionate (54%)	Collaborative (52%)
Collaborative (50%)	Calm (48%)
Kind (48%)	Compassionate (44%)
Calm (47%)	Humble (44%)

Exhibit 17: Gender of Leaders with Positive Influence (by Respondent Gender)

Respondent Gender	Female Leader	Male Leader	Total
Female	265 (64%)	149 (36%)	414 (100%)
Male	48 (30%)	110 (70%)	158 (100%)
Total	313	259	572

Exhibit 18: Traits of Successful Leaders (by Respondent Gender)

Traits	Female Respondents	Male Respondents
Accountable	264 (64%)	102 (64%)
Ambitious	163 (39%)	63 (40%)
Arrogant	8 (2%)	5 (3%)
Blames others	3 (1%)	2 (1%)
Calm	171 (41%)	57 (36%)
Charismatic	107 (26%)	52 (33%)

Exhibit 18: Traits of Successful Leaders (by Respondent Gender) *(continued)*

Traits	Female Respondents	Male Respondents
Collaborative	212 (51%)	98 (62%)
Compassionate	170 (41%)	54 (34%)
Condescending	9 (2%)	4 (3%)
Dishonest	7 (2%)	0 (0%)
Empathetic	75 (18%)	22 (14%)
Generous	127 (31%)	39 (25%)
Harsh	16 (4%)	4 (3%)
Holds others accountable	200 (48%)	77 (48%)
Humble	118 (28%)	54 (34%)
Inconsiderate	10 (2%)	1 (1%)
Insensitive	8 (2%)	4 (3%)
Kind	162 (39%)	59 (37%)
Passive	24 (6%)	7 (4%)
Self-focused	56 (14%)	28 (18%)

Exhibit 19: Top Five Traits of Successful Leaders (by Respondent Gender)

Female Respondents	Male Respondents
Accountable (64%)	Accountable (64%)
Collaborative (51%)	Collaborative (62%)
Holds others accountable (48%)	Holds others accountable (48%)
Calm (41%)	Ambitious (40%)
Compassionate (41%)	Kind (37%)

Exhibit 20: Gender of Successful Leaders (by Respondent Gender)

Respondent Gender	Female Leader	Male Leader	Total
Female	250 (61%)	163 (40%)	413 (100%)
Male	45 (29%)	112 (71%)	157 (100%)
Total	**295**	**275**	**570**

Exhibit 21: Traits of Leaders with Negative Influence (by Respondent Gender)

Traits	Female Respondents	Male Respondents
Accountable	18 (4%)	6 (4%)
Ambitious	62 (15%)	21 (20%)
Arrogant	212 (51%)	88 (55%)
Blames others	204 (49%)	83 (52%)
Calm	19 (5%)	10 (6%)
Charismatic	29 (7%)	9 (6%)
Collaborative	8 (2%)	6 (4%)
Compassionate	7 (2%)	2 (1%)
Condescending	210 (51%)	79 (50%)
Dishonest	145 (35%)	56 (35%)
Empathetic	13 (3%)	5 (3%)
Generous	8 (2%)	6 (4%)
Harsh	161 (39%)	54 (34%)
Holds others accountable	69 (17%)	21 (13%)
Humble	6 (1%)	5 (3%)
Inconsiderate	214 (51%)	77 (48%)
Insensitive	199 (48%)	66 (42%)
Kind	11 (3%)	6 (4%)
Passive	54 (13%)	21 (13%)
Self-focused	192 (46%)	76 (48%)

Exhibit 22: Top Five Traits of Leaders with Negative Influence (by Respondent Gender)

Female Respondents	Male Respondents
Arrogant (51%)	Arrogant (55%)
Condescending (51%)	Blames others (52%)
Inconsiderate (51%)	Condescending (50%)
Blames others (49%)	Inconsiderate (48%)
Insensitive (48%)	Self-focused (48%)

Exhibit 23: Gender of Leaders with Negative Influence (by Respondent Gender)

Respondent Gender	Female Leader	Male Leader	Total
Female	233 (56%)	180 (43%)	413 (100%)
Male	61 (38%)	98 (62%)	159 (100%)
Total	294	278	572

Exhibit 24: Traits of Unsuccessful Leaders (by Respondent Gender)

Traits	Female Respondents	Male Respondents
Accountable	14 (3%)	8 (5%)
Ambitious	49 (12%)	21 (13%)
Arrogant	186 (45%)	56 (35%)
Blames others	203 (49%)	91 (57%)
Calm	51 (12%)	16 (10%)
Charismatic	24 (6%)	12 (8%)

(continued)

Exhibit 24: Traits of Unsuccessful Leaders (by Respondent Gender) *(continued)*

Traits	Female Respondents	Male Respondents
Collaborative	12 (3%)	9 (6%)
Compassionate	23 (6%)	8 (5%)
Condescending	149 (36%)	55 (35%)
Dishonest	127 (31%)	53 (33%)
Empathetic	26 (6%)	5 (3%)
Generous	24 (6%)	10 (6%)
Harsh	126 (30%)	44 (28%)
Holds others accountable	53 (13%)	19 (12%)
Humble	16 (4%)	12 (8%)
Inconsiderate	192 (46%)	56 (35%)
Insensitive	162 (39%)	66 (42%)
Kind	49 (12%)	14 (9%)
Passive	108 (26%)	49 (31%)
Self-focused	178 (43%)	76 (48%)

Exhibit 25: Top Five Traits of Unsuccessful Leaders (by Respondent Gender)

Female Respondents	Male Respondents
Blames others (49%)	Blames others (57%)
Inconsiderate (46%)	Self-focused (48%)
Arrogant (45%)	Insensitive (42%)
Self-focused (43%)	Arrogant (35%)
Insensitive (39%)	Condescending (35%)

Exhibit 26: Gender of Unsuccessful Leaders (by Respondent Gender)

Respondent Gender	Female Leader	Male Leader	Total
Female	200 (49%)	206 (51%)	406
Male	76 (48%)	82 (52%)	158
Total	276	288	564

I also conducted the following analyses by age group in order to better understand differences between different generations. The following tables summarize these findings.

Exhibit 27: Top Five Traits of Leaders with Positive Influence (by Age Group)

18–34 years	35–54 years	55–74 years
Compassionate (52%)	Accountable (59%)	Accountable (68%)
Accountable (50%)	Calm (50%)	Collaborative (59%)
Kind (45%)	Collaborative (50%)	Compassionate (55%)
Generous (42%)	Compassionate (50%)	Calm (51%)
Humble (42%)	Kind (47%)	Holds others accountable (48%)

Exhibit 28: Top Five Traits of Successful Leaders (by Age Group)

18–34 years	35–54 years	55–74 years
Accountable (58%)	Accountable (63%)	Accountable (69%)
Collaborative (52%)	Collaborative (54%)	Collaborative (56%)
Ambitious (43%)	Holds others accountable (50%)	Holds others accountable (52%)
Holds others accountable (38%)	Calm (41%)	Calm (41%)
Generous (38%)	Compassionate (40%)	Compassionate (49%)

Exhibit 29: Top Five Traits of Leaders with Negative Influence (by Age Group)

18–34 years	35–54 years	55–74 years
Blames others (60%)	Arrogant (54%)	Condescending (69%)
Arrogant (51%)	Inconsiderate (51%)	Inconsiderate (51%)
Inconsiderate (46%)	Condescending (50%)	Arrogant (50%)
Self-focused (45%)	Self-focused (47%)	Insensitive (50%)
Harsh (43%)	Insensitive (47%)	Blames others (50%)

Exhibit 30: Top Five Traits of Unsuccessful Leaders (by Age Group)

18–34 years	35–54 years	55–74 years
Blames others (52%)	Blames others (53%)	Self-focused (51%)
Inconsiderate (48%)	Inconsiderate (43%)	Blames others (48%)
Arrogant (47%)	Insensitive (42%)	Arrogant (42%)
Insensitive (45%)	Self-focused (42%)	Inconsiderate (41%)
Self-focused (42%)	Arrogant (41%)	Insensitive (40%)

About the Author

Amer Kaissi, PhD, joined the faculty of Trinity University in 2003 after earning a doctorate in health services research, policy, and administration from the University of Minnesota and a master of public health in hospital administration from the American University of Beirut in his native Lebanon. At Trinity, Dr. Kaissi teaches courses in institutional healthcare management, healthcare strategic planning and marketing, and healthcare human resources management, and he also directs the executive program. He has published numerous journal articles on leadership, convenient care and retail clinics, strategic planning, and quality of care and patient safety, and he is the author of *Flipping Healthcare Through Retail Clinics and Other Convenient Care Models* (IGI Global, 2015), a resource on new delivery models. Dr. Kaissi is a certified professional executive coach, working with healthcare administrators and physicians to maximize their leadership potential, and he also advises hospitals and physician practices on strategic and business planning and marketing projects.